# Praise for *Boundless Kitchen*

"Ben brings his unique spin on health and performance through a collection of beautiful, healthy, and tasty recipes unlike most others you may have encountered previously. Despite all the debate and uncertainties that prevail in navigating the world of food, Ben helps readers restore logic and style to the everyday activity of eating."

— **William Davis, M.D.**, #1 *New York Times* best-selling author of the Wheat Belly series, *Undoctored*, and *Super Gut*

"For a mostly anti-foodie like me—that is, someone who still wants evidence-based maximum performance out of what I eat with completely minimal fuss—Ben has written a really tasty book. Great science. Great writing."

— **Steven Kotler**, *New York Times* best-selling author and executive director of the Flow Research Collective

"Boundless means living without limits . . . If you are looking for limitless energy, health, and how to live your best life, this book is for you."

— **JJ Virgin**, triple-board certified nutrition expert and Fitness Hall of Famer

"No one does a deep dive into human health and performance like Ben Greenfield. He leaves no stone unturned as he explores all the recent (and ancient) science surrounding optimal health."

— **Mark Sisson**, founder of Primal Kitchen foods, *New York Times* best-selling author, and publisher of *Mark's Daily Apple*

"As someone who cares deeply about the quality of my food yet has zero interest in fad diets, *Boundless Kitchen* is the perfect recipe. It solves the dilemma of dogmatic eating, complicated cooking, and bland 'healthy' taste in one fell swoop. I couldn't find a single subpar ingredient in the entire book. Plus, the gorgeous photography also serves as a mouth-watering appetite stimulant. If you want to prepare the healthiest and most delicious food in the comfort of your own home, this is the book for you."

— **Luke Storey**, writer, meditation and metaphysics teacher, lifestyle design expert, and host of *The Life Stylist Podcast*

"Ben is the 'pointy end of the spear' when it comes to all things performance, health, and longevity. In addition to his encyclopedic theoretical base, Ben has the practical application of these topics dialed in, and this is perhaps best-represented by his new cookbook. Managing our nutrition is arguably the most important feature of our overall well-being and this is a phenomenal resource."

— **Robb Wolf**, former research biochemist and two-time *New York Times* and *Wall Street Journal* best-selling author of *The Paleo Solution* and *Wired to Eat*

"Ben has magically brought his incredible knowledge of biohacking, supplementation, and physical and spiritual development to the field of nutrition with this awesome new cookbook. Reclaim the fun and functional in fueling with *Boundless Kitchen*!"

— **Mark Divine**, founder and CEO of SEALFIT, *New York Times* best-selling author, and philanthropist

"*Boundless Kitchen* could easily be called *The Boundless Medicine Chest*, for as Hippocrates said, 'Food is man's best medicine.' Free of diet dogmas, Ben Greenfield's *Boundless Kitchen* opens us to a natural menu of ways to really enjoy food and let our meals be a source of nutrition, vitality, joy, and connection to nature and each other. When we treat nature with Love, she indeed offers us Her Boundless Kitchen."

— **Paul Chek**, holistic health practitioner and founder of the CHEK Institute

"Prepare to have your perspectives on food entirely transformed as *Boundless Kitchen* redefines the very essence of how food can fuel not just the body but also life's journey, igniting happiness along the way."

— Yuri Elkaim, nutrition, fitness, and fat loss expert and *New York Times* best-selling author

"If I was stuck on an island for the rest of my life and could only bring two things . . . one would be my wife . . . another would be Ben's cookbook."

— Joe De Sena, CEO and founder of Spartan and the Death Race and *New York Times* best-selling author of *Spartan Up*

"Ben's *Boundless Kitchen* cookbook offers amazing flavors and satisfying textures. Not only can these recipes transform your health, they will change your perception of what healthy eating can be . . . delicious!"

— Elle Russ, best-selling author of *The Paleo Thyroid Solution*

"Ben has managed to make an original, delicious, and relatively simple cookbook for eating in a way that will make you feel Boundless. Just when you think you've tried it all, this cookbook offers a creative take on science-backed superfoods. I highly recommend adding it to your kitchen and savoring your new creations."

— Emily Fletcher, founder of Ziva and author of *Stress Less, Accomplish More*

"Ben is always ahead of the game . . . Food first when it comes to investing in your longevity."

— Dr. Tamsin Lewis, founder and medical director of Wellgevity

"Rather than giving you some dogmatic diet and strict food rules, Ben Greenfield instead shows you how to expertly weave together superfoods, little-known kitchen tactics, nutrition density, digestibility, and many other important concepts in one easy-to-read cookbook that makes healthy eating fun again!"

— Dr. Daniel Pompa, global leader in health and wellness, author of *Cellular Healing Diet* and *Beyond*, and host of the *Cellular Healing TV* podcast and YouTube show

"Ben masterfully combines biohacking, flavor, food, and nutrition science to make eating healthy, fun, and shockingly good."

— Michelle Norris, CEO of Paleo f(x)™

"This cookbook, *Boundless Kitchen*, will totally reinvent the way you think about how food fuels the body, fuels your life, and fuels your happiness."

— Jason Wachob, founder and co-CEO of mindbodygreen

"WARNING: This recipe book will satisfy your tastebuds and make you healthier. LOL. All kidding aside . . . Ben is a foodie and a health nut and he's combined the healthiest foods in the tastiest ways. Bravo, Ben!"

— Matt Gallant, co-founder and CEO of BIOptimizers

# BOUNDLESS
## KITCHEN

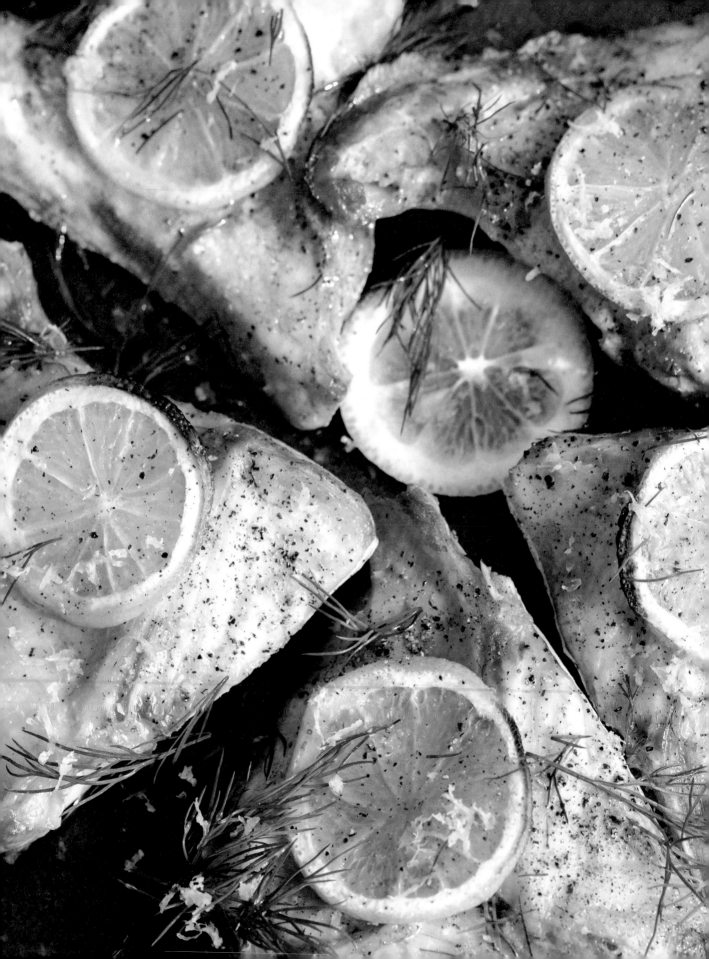

# BOUNDLESS
# KITCHEN

## BIOHACK YOUR BODY & BOOST YOUR BRAIN WITH HEALTHY RECIPES YOU ACTUALLY WANT TO EAT

# BEN GREENFIELD

**HAY HOUSE, INC.**
Carlsbad, California • New York City
London • Sydney • New Delhi

*Published in the United States by:* Hay House, Inc.: www.hayhouse.com®
• *Published in Australia by:* Hay House Australia Pty. Ltd.: www.hayhouse
.com.au • *Published in the United Kingdom by:* Hay House UK, Ltd.: www
.hayhouse.co.uk • *Published in India by:* Hay House Publishers India: www
.hayhouse.co.in

*Cover and interior design:* Karla Schweer • *Photography and food styling:* Sally
O'Neil @fitfoodieblog • *Cook:* Megan Yonsen • *Indexer:* Beverlee Day

**Cataloging-in-Publication Data is on file at the Library of Congress**

**Hardcover ISBN:** 978-1-4019-7773-3
**E-book ISBN:** 978-1-4019-7774-0

10  9  8  7  6  5  4  3  2  1
1st edition, November 2023
Printed in the United States of America

SUSTAINABLE
FORESTRY
INITIATIVE
Certified Chain of Custody
Promoting Sustainable Forestry
www.forests.org
SFI-01268
SFI label applies to the text stock

This product uses papers sourced from responsibly managed forests.
For more information, see www.hayhouse.com.

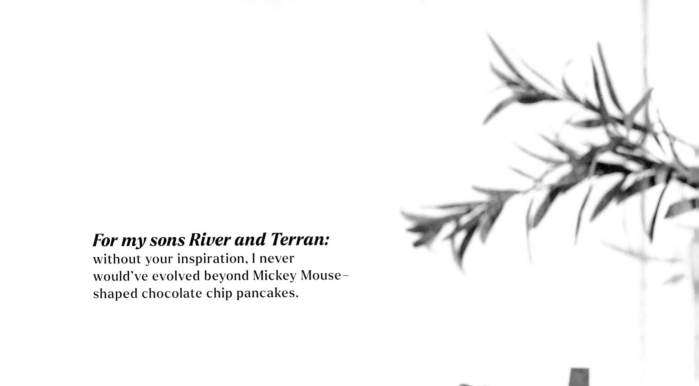

***For my sons River and Terran:***
without your inspiration, I never
would've evolved beyond Mickey Mouse–
shaped chocolate chip pancakes.

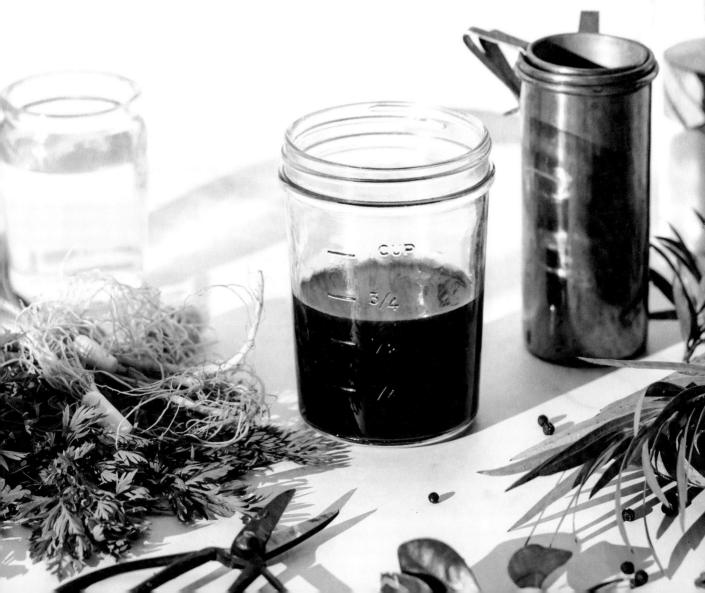

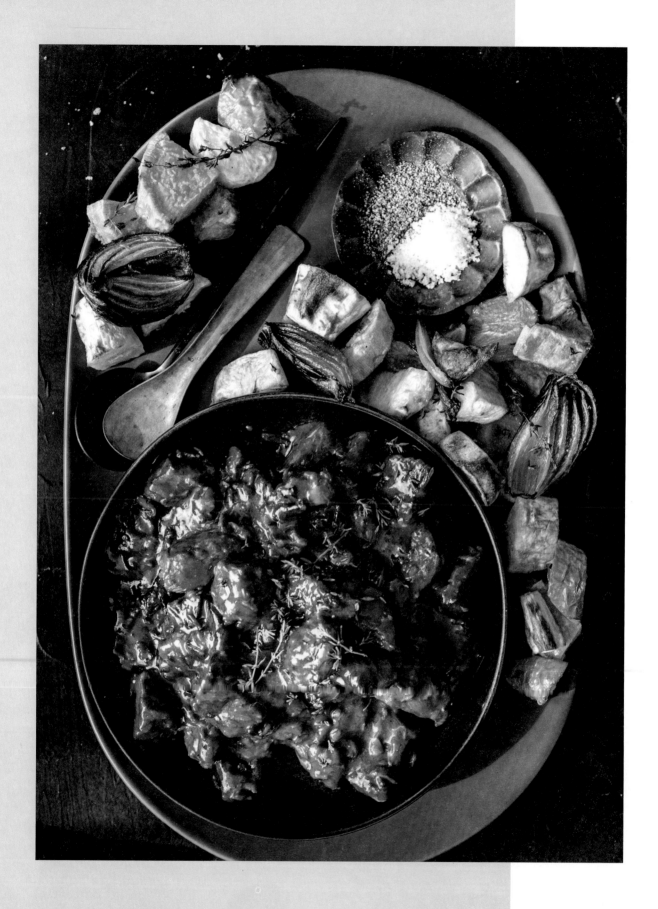

# Contents

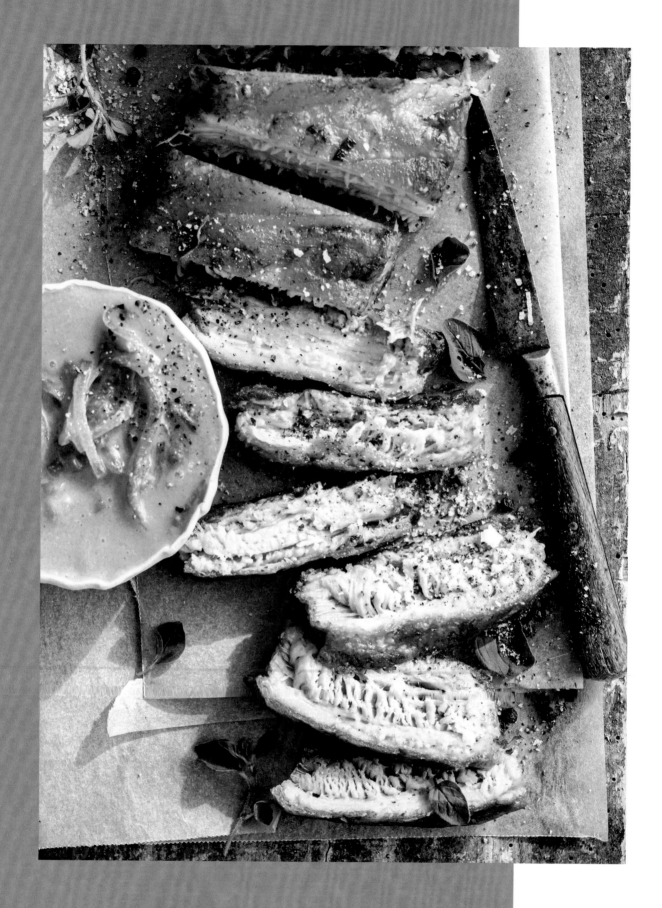

A few years ago, I told you in the opening pages of *Boundless Cookbook* that I was "not a chef." By most definitions of the word, I'm still not a chef, or a sous chef, or a line-order cook, or anything close to a professional culinary expert for that matter. I've never worked in a restaurant, never been paid to cook anything, never had a cooking show, never been on a cooking show, and would probably get lost, confused, and frustrated in the average commercial kitchen.

Instead, I'm just a biohacking nutritionist with a knack for food chemistry. I love to find unique ingredients and cooking methods from around the world and combine them in novel fashions to create recipes that haven't existed before. I look at conventional food and dishes and ask myself how I can maximize their healthful qualities—how can food provide me with all that clean, boundless energy I need in life? After all, I certainly agree with the idea that our food is what builds, cell by cell, our entire bodily structure, meaning that we are what we eat and we are what we eat *ate*. But as a guy with a master's degree in physiology, biomechanics, and nutrition, I also highly appreciate the fact that each of those tiny molecules of broken-down food that gets absorbed from your gut and transferred into your bloodstream serves as the very fuel that fires up every tiny muscle contraction, every brain neuron firing, and every goofy smile. So the way you look, feel, and perform every day of your life—for better or worse—

is directly influenced by the food on your fork. Crazy to think about, huh?

Perhaps it's because I'm *not* a classically trained chef that I'm able to somehow carve my own path in the kitchen and come up with recipes that most folks wouldn't think of, or at least wouldn't be stupid enough to try. In fact, I'd say I'm probably more of a mad scientist when it comes to food. I see colostrum and think it's not just for newborn babies but instead a welcome and creamy addition to a blueberry superfood smoothie. I dream up breakfast burritos with nutritious organ meats as their base. And I salivate over the idea of beef tongue tacos for dinner on a Tuesday.

These are meals you probably aren't going to find anywhere else. The result of all this mad science is unconventional yet healthy and delicious food that is fun to create and helps you live a long time. And while my methods and ingredients might be a bit unique, my desire for nutritious, superfood-inspired dishes that are both healthful and tasty is, well, not.

When it came out a few years ago, somehow my first cookbook struck a chord among my readers. People actually began smearing spent coffee grounds on their pork chops, eating their lunchtime salads wrapped in a seaweed roll burrito-style, and (shocker!) even trying organ meats like liver for the first time once they learned how to actually make them taste good.

In the three years since that first cookbook debuted, I have learned about even more valuable and life-changing nutrition concepts and ingredients that I cannot wait to share with you in an entertaining and hands-on way. Thus, *Boundless Kitchen* was conceived.

*Boundless Kitchen* is a cookbook for everyone, from beginners to advanced foodies, and as such, the food preparation featured in these pages is fun and manageable for all readers. I avoid any semblance of a myopic, rule-filled diet and instead aim to thrill your taste buds whenever you're looking for something interesting, healthy, and pleasurable to shove down your gaping maw.

While they're broken into neat categories within these pages, the recipes in this book are meant to be mixed and matched to your heart's (and stomach's) desire. For example, in the morning, perhaps a Nature's Multivitamin Breakfast Burrito paired with a Cacao Charcoal Latte; for lunch, a bit of wild pesto on a homemade tortilla with smoked and spiced crispy chicken; and for dinner, a Shiso Shrub Fusion cocktail with Sous Vide Pork Belly with Vinegar Deglaze Sauce, accompanied by a Parmesan Squash Wedges side and topped off with Pumpkin Spice Colostrum Cake for dessert. Toss in a few Chocolate Chai Gummies for dessert and you've got a quite gratifying day planned in the culinary department, along with all the clean, boundless energy you'd ever want.

The recipes in this cookbook come from a variety of places: from yours truly, as well as from my superstar wife, Jessa (creator of the fan-favorite cinnamon rolls featured in my first cookbook); from my two boys, River and Terran, who are burgeoning creative cooks in their own right (seriously—check out their YouTube channel, Go Greenfields); and from the brains of my Ben Greenfield Life coaching group

(which includes physicians, nutritionists, dietitians, personal trainers, and more).

But before we jump into the recipes themselves, we must first establish a few boundless guidelines for eating.

# THE BOUNDLESS GUIDELINES & MINDSET

While I mentioned above that I avoid rule-filled diets, when it comes to eating, there *are* a few guidelines that I follow, and I recommend you do too. In observing "Blue Zones"—that is, physical places with a disproportionately high number of centenarians—throughout the world (think places like Okinawa, Nicoya, Sardinia, and more), food scientists have seen some distinct dietary patterns emerge. These patterns reflect nutritionally related trends that can drastically affect one's health—for better or worse. Furthermore, although it's the dark and dirty secret in the health and fitness industry that if you want to make a few bucks fast, you should write a diet book and subsequently declare that diet to be the ultimate diet for all of humankind, the fact is that *there is no one perfect diet.* Instead, there is a great deal of biochemical, microbiome, and genetic diversity among us humans that dictates that not everyone is going to respond to a carnivore or a ketogenic or a vegan or a cayenne-pepper-maple-syrup-hot-sauce-shoot-fire-out-your-butthole diet in the same way.

But, like I mentioned above, there are key patterns that emerge among long-lived humans, no matter their ratio of fat to carbohydrate to protein and no matter how much vegetables versus meat they eat. A few of those key practices, patterns, trends, habits, routines, or whatever you want to call them, include:

## Eat in a Parasympathetic State

The first pattern is to eat in a parasympathetic state, the parasympathetic nervous system being the "rest-and-digest" branch of your nervous system. In other words, sit when you eat. Why?

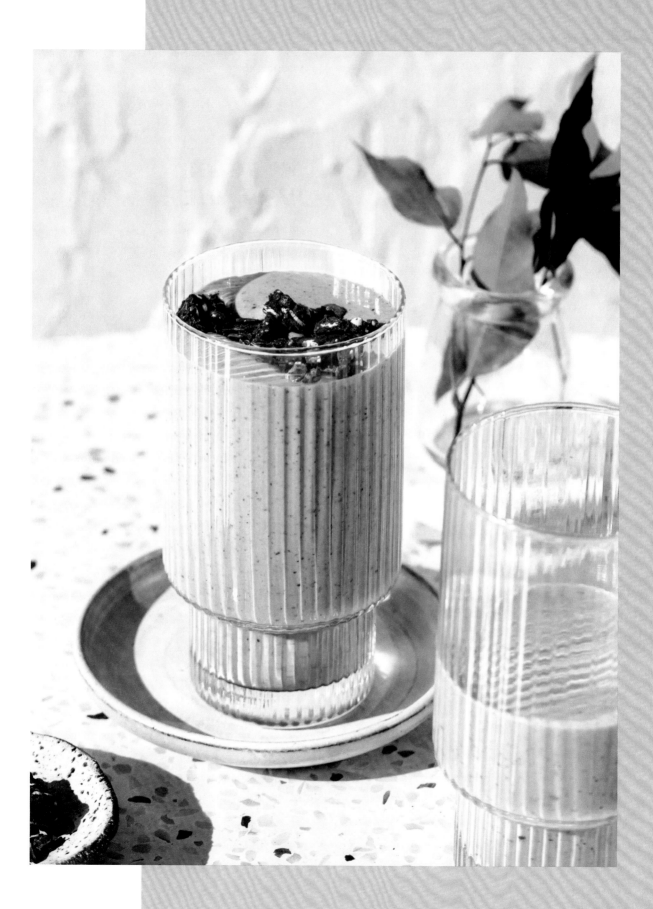

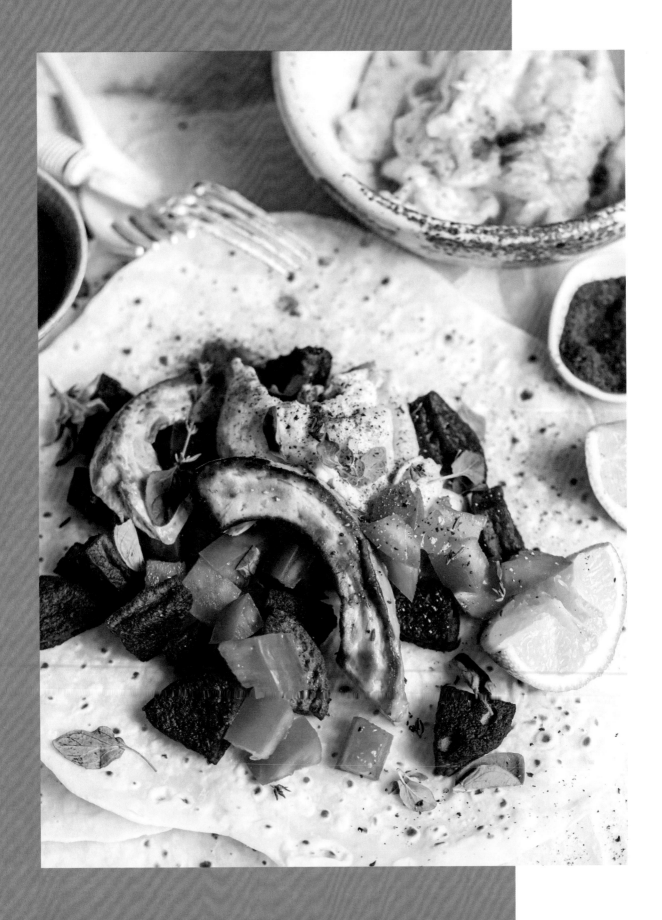

Simple: you'll digest your food better; experience less digestive distress, such as gas and bloating, from issues such as low enzyme production or so-called "leaky gut"; eat in a more mindful state; and feel fuller faster. To say it plainly, there's a notable difference between sipping on your superfood smoothie while you read the news, scroll through your favorite social media feed, or relax at your kitchen table, versus stressfully sucking down that same smoothie with one hand white-knuckled on a steering wheel as you blaze down the highway at 60 miles per hour during your morning commute. Eat in a relaxed, de-stressed state whenever possible; if you can't, well, just wait to eat. You won't starve—trust me. In addition, adopt some kind of gratitude or prayer practice before a meal. Pause, take a few relaxing breaths, thank God for your food, think of how grateful you are for your sustenance, and then open your eyes and eat, slowly.

## Eat with People

The longest human study on happiness to date—detailed in the excellent book *The Good Life: Lessons from the World's Longest Scientific Study of Happiness*—found that the top secret to a good life with an optimized health span and life span is not some expensive supplement or biohack or 5 A.M. sprint up the side of a steep mountain. Rather, the secret is in the quality of your friendships and relationships, and there's nothing that brings people together quite like sharing good food. Bread was meant to be broken together. Wine was meant to be sipped while laughing with a friend (don't snort it out your nose). Grandma's broccoli casserole (no matter how gassy it might make you) was meant to be consumed during memorable and heartwarming family gatherings, not while you're locked away in your bedroom closet during a midnight snack raid. Your dining room and living room (no matter how messy or small or cat hair–laden or embarrassing to you) were meant for dinner parties with friends in your local community. Families were meant to celebrate glorious dinners together as many nights of the week as possible, and sometimes waffles together for breakfast too.

So as much as you possibly can, share your meals with other human beings.

## Control Blood Glucose and Inflammation

Tossing your blood sugar levels onto a daily roller coaster adventure, a practice that produces something known as "high glycemic variability," can lead to the onset of a wide variety of chronic diseases, not to mention a rampant appetite, up-and-down energy levels that are anything but stable, and damage to fats within your blood vessels and other tissues. Inflammation from stress, poor sleep, environmental toxins, and high consumption of ultra-processed foods and vegetable oils can throw a few extra wrenches into your precious biology. I tell people that if there are just two biomarkers to track to see if you're going to live a long time, they would indeed be your blood sugar levels and your inflammation. But the good news is that you can take steps to control these factors. First, as I already stated, eat in a parasympathetic, relaxed state. In addition, to activate enzymes and hormones that help digest food and keep blood sugar stable, and also to limit dietary components such as processed ingredients and rancid fats that can lead to inflammation, you can:

- Chew each bite of food 25 to 40 times (yes, you can go back and read that again—I really do mean 25 to 40 times).

- Avoid eating out of packages and containers and from any sources that have been heavily processed, particularly making every attempt to limit or eliminate vegetable oils and hydrogenated oils such as canola oil, safflower oil, sunflower oil, margarine, and "fake," diluted non–extra virgin olive oil.

- Keep your eye out for the host of additives, preservatives, colorings, and other hard-to-metabolize materials so often found in packaged foods, even those notoriously marked as health food. Those bastards. They snuck canola oil, cane sugar, Red No. 40, Yellow

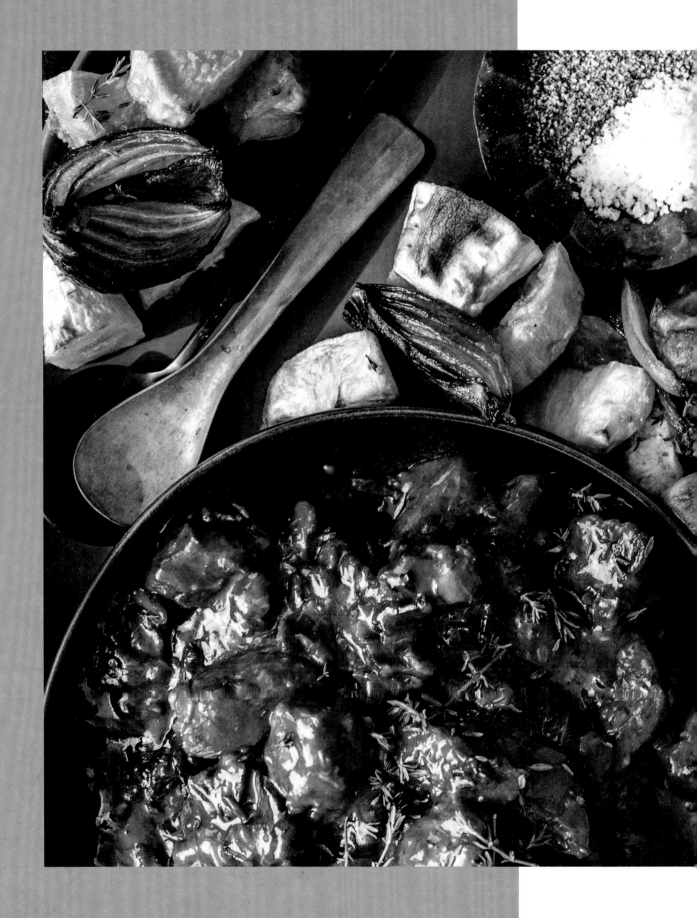

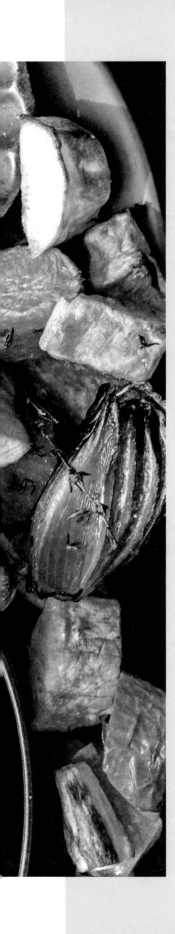

**Whenever possible, prepare your food slowly and mindfully.**

**"Buy-open-devour" is far inferior to "grow-soak-sprout-ferment-care-love-enjoy-savor."**

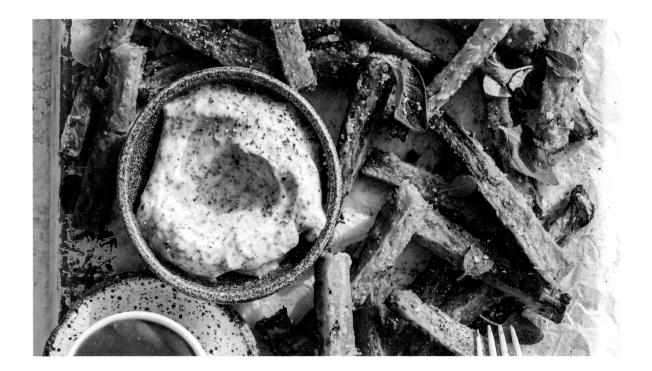

No. 5, and Yellow No. 6 into your nutty, "natural" trail mix again.

- Mitigate your sugar and starch consumption, and try to primarily consume carbs before, during, or after physical activity or after thermal stress such as heat or cold.

- Consume blood glucose disposal agents prior to a meal, such as apple cider vinegar, Ceylon cinnamon, berberine, bitter melon extract, or Backyard Bitters or a fantastic Shiso Shrub Fusion cocktail. (Hint: You'll find these on pages 99 and 89, respectively, in this cookbook.) In addition, spicy ingredients like cayenne and hot sauces have been shown to suppress hunger and increase satiety after a meal. So what that means is that you want to cook with plenty of sour (e.g., vinegar), bitter (e.g., bitter melon), and spicy (e.g., red pepper) ingredients if you want to control both blood glucose and hunger.

- Fast regularly, such as a daily 10- to 12-hour fast for women and a 12- to 16-hour fast for men (whoa, wait . . . you're telling me that females and males have differing biological responses to caloric restriction?). Consider a bi-monthly

24-hour dinner-to-dinner fast and a quarterly detox, such as a juice cleanse, a bone broth cleanse, or a fasting-mimicking diet in which you reduce your usual calorie intake considerably for several days. If you want to delve deeper into the topic of detox or cleanses, check out my book *Boundless*, in which I cover all this in exhaustive scientific detail.

## Eat Slowly and Intentionally

Finally, if you're anything like me and have a hard time actually pushing yourself away from the table without overstuffing yourself, or you constantly find yourself thinking about food between meals, then you should know that the best practical strategies that may support higher satiety levels—especially if you're restricting calories as some kind of a weight loss or longevity-enhancing strategy—include eating more slowly, avoiding hyper-palatable, ultra-processed, "soft" textured meals, and structuring each meal to include decent amounts of protein, fiber, and water content. Related to that last bit, this is why I'm a huge fan of low-calorie, high-water-content ingredients such as chia seed slurry, Japanese yam noodles, pumpkin mash, sea moss gel, smoothies blended thick with lots of ice, bone broth, and a few of the other "gel-like" foods you'll find within the pages of this cookbook. You'll feel like you're eating a decent amount of food, but you really aren't consuming very many calories at all when you include these types of compounds.

These four simple practices will put boundless energy from food at your beck and call.

Food enjoyment is also a mental mindset. To maximize the benefits of the Blue Zone practices previously listed, combine those four guidelines with these other mentalities:

- Whenever possible, prepare your food slowly and mindfully. "Buy-open-devour" is far inferior to "grow-soak-sprout-ferment-care-love-enjoy-savor." No, I'm not saying that every time you want to have yogurt you need to crush *L. reuteri* probiotic tablets with a mortar and pestle, combine them with raw goat's milk that has been boiled and cooled, and then ferment the mixture in a covered dish for 36 hours in your oven at low temperature (although that's a darn good way to make some of the best food ever for your gut). That would be exhausting. But is it asking too much for you to perhaps learn how to drench a lovely whole chicken in extra virgin olive oil and sea salt and throw it in the oven for 35 minutes instead of picking up a bucket of fried chicken on the way home from work, or grabbing the canola oil–drenched, factory-farmed rotisserie chicken from the grocery store?

- Be in constant awe of and gratitude for the wonders of God's creation, embracing cease-less curiosity about the magic, beauty, mys-tery, and wonder of the vast array of super-foods scattered across this earth and allowing yourself to go on a culinary adventure to try them. When you see ingredients like Barùkas nuts, Himalayan tartary buckwheat flour, maca root, and phytoplankton bloom minerals, don't be afraid to experiment with them (not in a reckless, eating-scary-things, TV show kind of way, but rather in a wise and discerning explo-ration of food kind of way).

- Consider food not as just a collection of physi-cal atoms and molecules largely disconnected from the ethereal dimensions of your spirit but as a means to fuel your soul. Remember that what you put into your body is important not only for your physical health but also for your spiritual health and, ultimately, for fulfilling your life's purpose. So, yes, mowing down a bag of potato chips at the movie theater or on the airplane or in front of your basement TV will make you far less capable of crushing the next day compared to munching on a few Brazil nuts along with some organic dark chocolate (gulp: did I just admit to being that guy who sneaks Brazil nuts into the movie theater?).

Tips, tips, tips: I'm tired of tips.

It's time to eat.

So allow me to finish this introduction with a quick but meaningful reminder from 1 Corinthians 10:31: *"So whether you eat or drink or whatever you do, do it all for the glory of God."*

Now, *mangia, mangia.* Let's eat.

*Ben Greenfield*

# Plants 'n' Roots

As you learned in the introduction to this cookbook, there is no "one size fits all" diet. But no matter what nutrition plan you follow, there are specific characteristics that are repeatedly seen in the diets of most of the healthiest and longest-living individuals on earth. They include incorporating fasting regularly, eating in a parasympathetic state via practices (such as chewing each bite thoroughly), engaging in relaxing conversation with friends and family during meals, and, quite notably, eating real food, as fresh and close to nature as possible, with a wide variety of proteins, fats, carbohydrates, plants, herbs, and spices, while avoiding vegetable oils, processed sugar, and acellular carbohydrates.

*For all resources, books, tools, and ingredients mentioned throughout this chapter, go to: BoundlessKitchen.com/resources*

Acellular carbohydrates? Huh? Allow me to explain.

*Cellular* plant foods have a low carbohydrate density compared to the *acellular* flour, sugar, and grains that are dominant in most Western diets. These acellular carbohydrates, due to heavier processing, lack intact cells, so they can raise your blood sugar faster and aren't as good for your gut microbiome—kind of like fast-burning kindling versus a slow-burning log. In contrast, roots and tubers (also known as USOs, or underground storage organs), fruits, leaves, stems, and the like all store their carbohydrates in fiber-walled living cells that are high in nutrients. These cells remain largely intact during cooking. This basically means that the maximum carbohydrate density they can have is quite low, they don't mess with your blood sugar levels as much, and they're more nutrient-dense. Higher carbohydrate density means that you get more carbs with fewer nutrients, and the carbohydrate density of acellular carbohydrates is about 75 percent, while that of cellular carbohydrates is closer to 25 percent. One study, entitled "Comparison with ancestral diets suggests dense acellular carbohydrates promote an inflammatory microbiota, and may be the primary dietary cause of leptin resistance and obesity," sums up the idea that consuming a larger amount of carrots, parsnips, beets, yucca, turnips, and potatoes, for example, is a pretty good idea when it comes to your overall carbohydrate intake.

Hence the idea of thinking of your vegetable and carbohydrate intake as a mix of eating plants 'n' roots. The result is higher nutrient density, better fuel for the gut bacteria, and fewer blood sugar roller coaster rides. Now don't get me wrong: I don't totally swear off acellular carbohydrates, especially a bit of overnight oatmeal with blueberries and fresh maple syrup or a slice of fermented sourdough bread with raw honey and sea salt, but the lion's share of my carbs truly is derived from cellular carbohydrates, which make up the majority of carbohydrates found in this cookbook.

Finally, you might be concerned about the newfangled, popular idea that plants have toxic, built-in defense mechanisms that can harm your gut, thus dictating you should eat only meat (a "carnivore diet"). While human beings can

survive—and some may argue, even *thrive*—solely on a nose-to-tail carnivore diet, the more important question is whether it is a scalable, sustainable option. My answer to that is: probably not. It is actually rare to find a long-lived, healthy population that subsists entirely on meat, especially muscle meat. For example, several Asian, Latin American, and African tribal cultures actually consume the intestines of ruminant animals like goats, sheep, deer, and cows; but they all contain high amounts of the vegetables and fiber that those animals consumed—a literal stomach salad!

Fact is, via many of the fermentation, soaking, sprouting, and food preparation methods you'll find within the pages of this book, you can deactivate plant defense mechanisms and render most plants, nuts, seeds, and herbs pretty darn digestible, especially if you aren't dealing with serious gut issues such as intestinal permeability, gastric inflammation, or diverticulitis.

I certainly have a "nose-to-tail" approach to eating meat, by including not just muscle meat but also organ meats, bone marrow, and bone broth. But I also include cooked, puréed, smashed, and blended root vegetables and tubers; homemade yogurt made from coconut or goat milk and probiotics; raw organic honey as a sweetener; small, antioxidant-rich, low-sugar berries such as blueberries and blackberries; bitter and tannin-rich beverages such as organic wine, teas, and coffees; seeds and nuts that have been soaked, fermented, or sprouted; nutrient-dense vegetable powders that offer plenty of phytonutrients without excess roughage and fiber; and some, but not much, raw roughage, such as spring mix salads or sprouts in my smoothie.

I'm often asked if I still have a "big-ass salad" for lunch, as I've mentioned a few times in the past on my podcast. Here's the thing: I *do* tend to eat a lot of mashed, pureed, cooked, fermented, and otherwise leftover vegetables with most lunches, along with a giant cup of bone broth and usually some chopped avocados and small cold-water fish like sardines or anchovies, but I no longer consume oodles of raw roughage in the form of giant piles of kale, spinach, and greens. I've found this

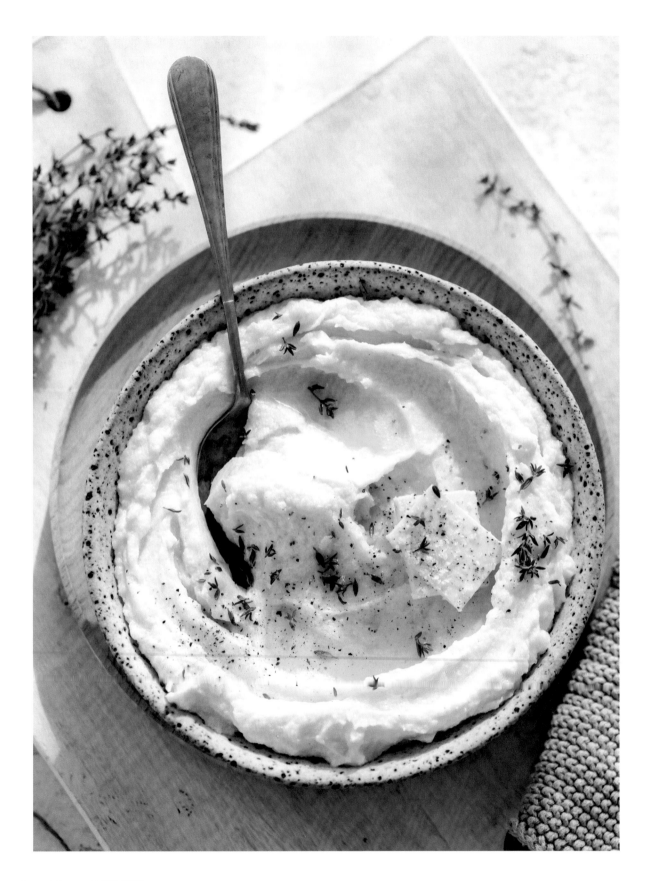

to be far friendlier for my gut, particularly when it comes to limiting bloating and digestion. For most such lunches, I wrap up all these plants and roots either "burrito-style"—in a dark-green, nutrient-packed seaweed nori sheet, a rice paper roll that I soak in warm water for about 30 seconds—or open-faced sandwich style on top of a few giant slices of fresh tomato and/or cucumber. As a matter of fact, I'm now nearly incapable of enjoying a salad with a standard fork and much prefer eating my vegetables as a burrito or on a tomato/cucumber bread-free sandwich. Try it sometime!

# What about Carnivorous Ancestral Populations?

Many will argue of the existence of carnivorous ancestral populations. While it's true that some of our ancestors thrived on large quantities of animal products, every single one of the commonly cited carnivorous groups also took significant advantage of plant foods. For example:

**The nomads of Mongolia** ate plenty of meat and dairy products but consumed wild onions and garlic, tubers and roots, seeds, and berries.

**Gaucho Brazilians** consumed mostly beef but also supplemented their diet with yerba mate, a tea rich in vitamins, minerals, and phytonutrients.

**The Maasai, Rendille, and Samburu tribes of East Africa** primarily consumed meat, milk, and blood but also occasionally ate herbs and tree barks. Women and older men in these communities consumed ample amounts of fruit, tubers, and honey.

**The Russian Arctic Chukotka** thrived on fish, caribou, and marine animals but always paired these animal foods with local roots, leafy greens, berries, or seaweed.

**The Sioux of South Dakota** ate large amounts of buffalo but also consumed wild fruit, nuts, and seeds that they came across as they hunted the buffalo herds.

**The Canadian Inuit** subsisted primarily on walrus, whale meat, seal, and fish but also foraged wild berries, lichens, and sea vegetables and even fermented many of these plant foods as a preservation method.

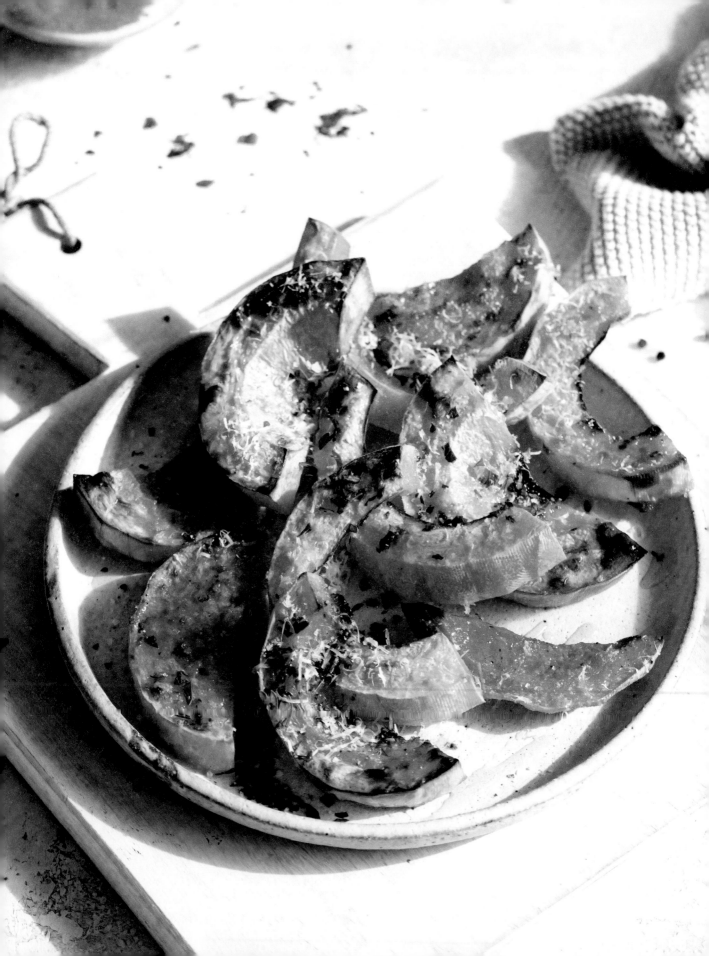

# Parmesan Squash Wedges

*Yield:* 4 SERVINGS (ABOUT 20 WEDGES)

*Total Time:* 55 MINUTES

**TOOLS AND MATERIALS**

Baking sheet

Parchment paper

**INGREDIENTS**

1 medium-size butternut squash (but you can substitute sweet potatoes if you like), peeled, de-seeded and cut into "half-moons," about ½ inch thick.

⅛ cup extra-virgin olive oil or, for more heat stability, avocado oil

Salt and black pepper, to taste

¼ cup grated Parmigiano-Reggiano cheese

1 whole nutmeg, grated, or 1 tablespoon nutmeg powder

My wife, Jessa, often whips up these wedges to go along with an evening meal of roast chicken, broiled fish, or grilled steak. The crisp saltiness of the baked Parmesan combined with the luscious softness of the oiled squash easily place this recipe in the same coveted category as another of my wife's specialties: bacon-wrapped dates. But we'll save those dates for another day (see page 16) and focus here on the wedges, which I personally love to sprinkle with a bit of coarse salt and dip in Primal Kitchen ketchup or buffalo sauce.

Incidentally, if you prefer to eat dairy-free, you can simply bake the squash without the Parmesan cheese and then sprinkle it with nutritional yeast, ground cashews, garlic powder, and salt. This mix is a good alternative to cheese and still gives the recipe the nice umami flavor that pairs well with the sweetness of the squash. If you do use Parmesan, then technically you should try to choose actual Parmigiano-Reggiano cheese, which is the real deal with superior flavor, longer aging time, and better ingredients. For true, traditional Parmigiano-Reggiano cheese, just three ingredients are used: the highest quality raw cow's milk, animal rennet (enzymes from mammalian stomach), and salt.

1. Preheat oven to 375°F.

2. Line a baking sheet with parchment paper and spread the squash half-moons on the sheet, making sure none of the squash pieces are stacked on top of each other.

3. Drizzle the olive or avocado oil over the squash and lightly salt/pepper it (but don't be heavy handed; remember, the Parmigiano is already a salty cheese).

4. Roast for 30 to 40 minutes, or until the squash can be easily penetrated with a fork.

5. Remove from oven, set oven to broil, and then generously sprinkle the Parmigiano on top of all the squash pieces.

6. Place the cheese-topped squash back into the oven about 6 to 8 inches from broiler and broil until the cheese is golden-brown (about 3 to 5 minutes—watch carefully to avoid burning).

7. Remove the squash from the oven and then grate nutmeg all over the squash (nutmeg is a very potent spice so go easy on it). Serve.

# Bacon-Wrapped, Almond-Stuffed Dates

*Yield:* 4 SERVINGS

*Total Time:* 50 TO 60 MINUTES

**TOOLS AND MATERIALS**

Toothpicks

Baking sheet

**INGREDIENTS**

15 to 20 pitted Medjool dates

30 to 40 salted roasted almonds

1-pound pack of pasture-raised bacon

Yes, yes, I know: most folks will drool about bacon-wrapped *anything*. But you'll swear you've gone to appetizer heaven once you've popped a few of these soft, sweet dates wrapped in salty, smoky bacon and baked to crispy-soft perfection, with the sweet, soft crunch of an almond in the center. This dish is another of my wife's specialties and is a big hit for any dinner party. It is also a traditional staple of our Christmas Eve appetizer feast, which often also includes homemade Thai chicken wraps, chicken skewers with peanut sauce, a charcuterie board with select meats and cheeses, and fresh eggnog dusted with cinnamon.

When I smell the sugary dates and smoky-bacon aromas wafting up from the kitchen, I know Jessa is planning on packing an extra pound on my waistline during that evening's dinner. So yes, enjoy these addictively good treats, but in moderation; I usually "allow" myself two to four bacon-wrapped dates, after which I suspect the combo of fat, protein, and sugar is probably a bit too much for my cells to handle.

You can use any dates you'd like for this recipe, but I recommend Medjool. Native to Morocco, Medjool dates are just one of hundreds of date varieties, but they're the variety known as "the fruit of kings" because they were originally eaten by royalty as a tactic to fight off fatigue. Medjool dates have a sweet caramel taste and chewy texture and, like many other dates, are high in fiber, potassium, magnesium, copper, antioxidants, and vitamin B.

1. Preheat the oven to 350°F.

2. Stuff each date with 1 to 2 almonds.

3. Cut the bacon into 2½-inch pieces.

4. Wrap the stuffed dates with bacon, secure them with a toothpick, and lay them seam side down on the baking sheet.

5. Bake for 30 to 45 minutes, turning halfway through so the bacon is evenly cooked, until the bacon is crispy.

6. Serve warm or at room temperature.

***Fun fact:*** In Britain, bacon-wrapped dates are traditionally called "Devils on Horseback," either due to their devilish black and red coloring, the fact that they serve as a counterpart to another British dish called Angels on Horseback (bacon-wrapped oysters), or the substantial amount of cayenne pepper called for in the original Devils on Horseback recipe, which makes them "devilishly" hot. Or perhaps they get their name for all three reasons.

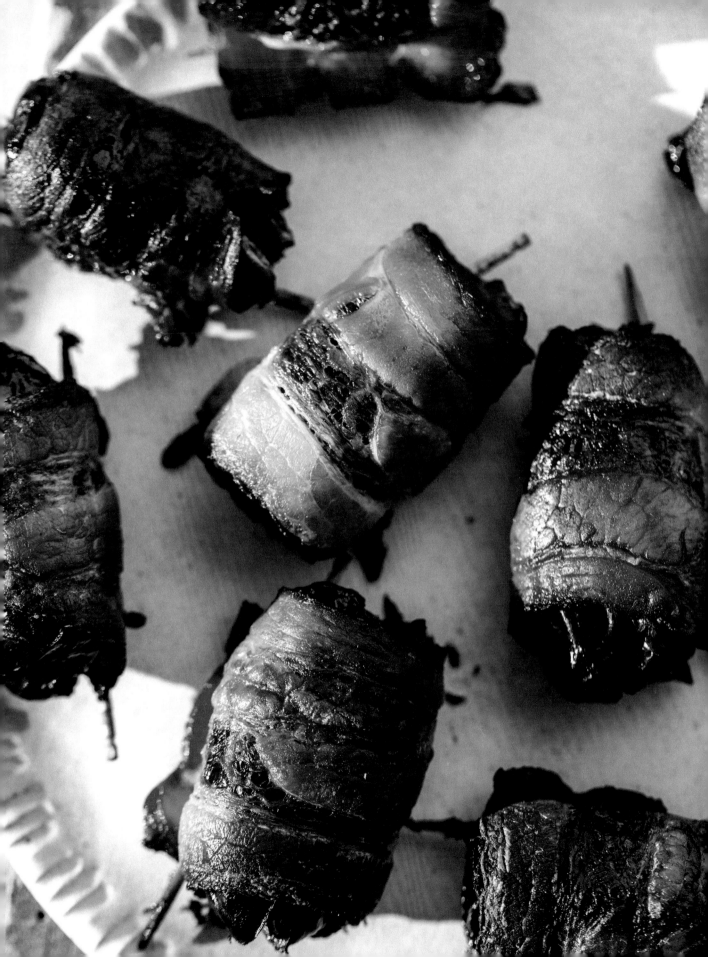

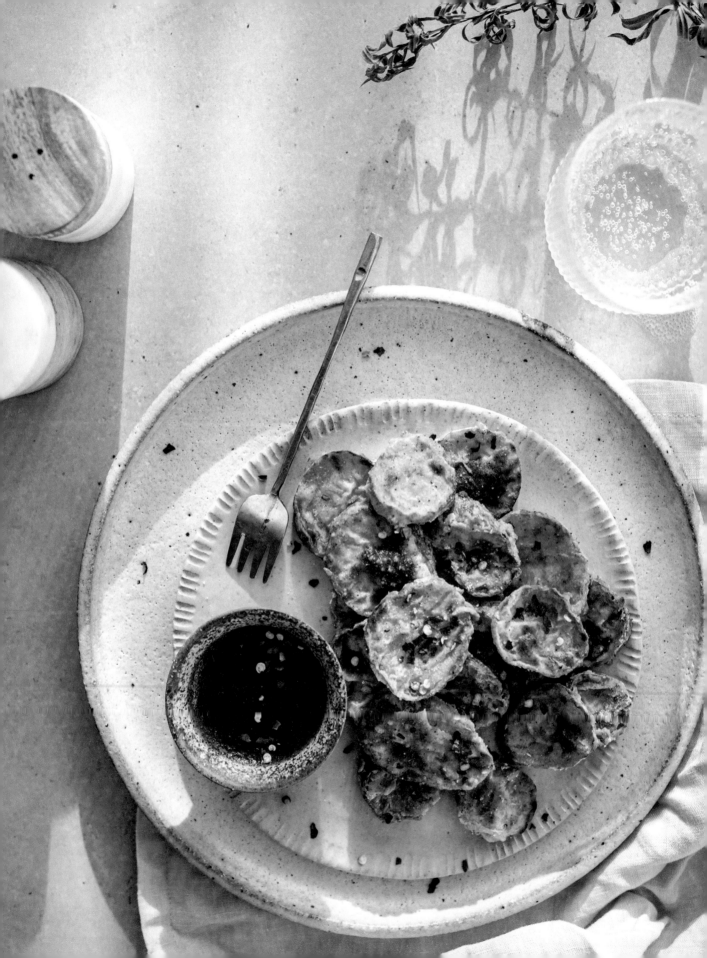

# Air-Fried Pickles

This recipe gives you a crunchy, salty, low-calorie snack or side dish with minimal prep time and is a great alternative to popcorn. It is an enjoyable snack to accompany any cocktail or glass of wine or beer. I like to dip mine in a bit of Joey's Hot Sauce or Primal Kitchen mustard, ketchup, or (highly recommended) buffalo sauce.

1. Preheat the air fryer to 375°F.

2. In a small bowl, mix together the flour, tapioca starch, and spices. In a separate bowl, whisk the egg.

3. Dry the pickles well on a towel to remove any excess moisture. Spray the air fryer basket with avocado oil.

4. Dip a pickle slice into the beaten egg and then dredge in the flour mixture. Place the breaded pickle in the air fryer basket.

5. Repeat with the remaining pickles. Lightly mist the tops of the pickles with avocado oil spray or drizzle lightly with olive oil.

6. Place the basket into the air fryer for about 10 to 12 minutes, or until the outside of the pickle slice is golden brown. Allow them to cool slightly before removing them from the basket.

*Yield:* 3 TO 4 SERVINGS

*Total Time:* 20 MINUTES

**TOOLS AND MATERIALS**

Air fryer

**INGREDIENTS**

¼ cup almond or other gluten-free flour

2 tablespoons tapioca starch

¾ teaspoon onion powder

½ teaspoon garlic powder

½ teaspoon paprika

½ teaspoon black pepper

¼ teaspoon salt

¼ teaspoon turmeric

1 medium or large egg

1 cup sliced pickles

Avocado oil spray or extra virgin olive oil

**Note:** *Breville and Cuisinart are two good brands of air fryers. For more on brands, go to BoundlessKitchen.com/resources.*

## AIR FRYERS

When I published *Boundless Cookbook*, I was right on the cusp of shopping for my first air fryer, but never had a chance to experiment in time for the book to include any air fryer recipes. Nonetheless, I was intrigued with this method of cooking, which can produce a crisp, golden crust similar to deep-fat frying but without all the unhealthy oils and fat oxidation. Basically, air fryers contain a fan that circulates hot air at high speed, just like a miniature countertop convection oven.

As a result of this mechanism, just a tiny amount of cooking oil is needed compared to standard frying. Air fryers also significantly reduce cooking time and tend to give off less heat, which makes them ideal for whipping up a quick recipe on the kitchen countertop. They are an extra cooking tool should your oven be full of other items, which is often the case in our house if we happen to be preparing meat in the oven, but want to make some kind of a side dish. Air fryers are incredibly versatile because you can use them not only for frying but also for things like roasting vegetables, cooking meats, or baking cookies. Some manufacturers, like Breville, even offer handy "multi cookers" that combine an air fryer, toaster oven, and pressure cooker all in one.

# Air-Fried Roots 'n' Tubers

Whether you are limiting your carb intake and feel like standard potato fries might pack too hefty a starch punch, or you need a creative use for all those extra tubers (such as carrots) that you might have in the fridge, look no further. Enter the air-fried root or tuber.

Root vegetables are nutrient-dense cellular carbohydrates with a relatively low sugar content and, when prepared in the right way, can deliver all the flavor of French fries but with no vegetable oil, relatively fewer carbs, and, when prepared in an air fryer, much less heat damage to the fragile fats in plant oils you use in your recipe. Who knew fresh carrots were such a good substitute for greasy potatoes?

And it's not just carrots. From parsnips and turnips to sweet potatoes and taro to zucchini and butternut squash, the combinations of roots and tubers you can air fry are endless, with dozens of shape, spice, topping, and dipping options.

The basic instructions below can be applied to just about any root or tuber. The cooking time will vary depending on whether you use an air fryer or an oven, as well as the thickness and density of your chosen ingredient and whether you thin slice, thick slice, sideways slice, or cube it. Cooking times also vary depending on whether you prefer a steak-fry style tenderness or (like I do) a golden, lightly browned, crunchy texture.

1. Preheat the air fryer or oven to 400°F. Wash and peel the roots or tubers and then cut them into even-size sticks, slices, or cubes of your preferred size. I typically cut pieces about 1 inch thick.

2. Put the cut ingredients into a large bowl and sprinkle the flour (if using) and all the spices (including the cayenne, if using) over them until they're thoroughly coated.

3. Drizzle the extra virgin olive oil over everything, and stir or toss in the bowl to evenly coat with the oil.

4. Place the roots or tubers on the air fryer pan or on a baking sheet lined with parchment paper. Make sure they are evenly spread and not stacked on top of each other.

5. Air fry or bake for 20 to 35 minutes. (Air frying will be on the shorter end of this range; baking will take slightly longer.) Check them halfway through to move them around or flip/toss them to make sure they cook evenly.

6. Your dish is done when there is a slight browning or crisping on the edges and/or you can pierce the roots or tubers easily with a fork.

7. Remove the roots or tubers from the oven or fryer, and let them cool for a couple of minutes before serving.

*Yield:* 4 SERVINGS

*Total Time:* VARIES, BUT USUALLY 20 TO 35 MINUTES

**TOOLS AND MATERIALS**

Air fryer or oven

Parchment paper

**INGREDIENTS**

1 pound roots or tubers of your choice

2 tablespoons gluten-free flour, such as coconut, breadfruit, or arrowroot (optional)

1 teaspoon salt of your choice

½ teaspoon black pepper

½ teaspoon garlic powder

½ teaspoon onion powder

½ teaspoon dried thyme

½ teaspoon cayenne powder (optional)

2 tablespoons extra virgin olive oil or avocado oil spray

**Notes:** *While the flour is optional, it can lend some nice added texture and flavor. For more kick, add the cayenne. Of course, you can experiment with any spices you like, such as dill, paprika, or even cinnamon, cacao, and honey. For more on my favorite salts, check out BoundlessKitchen.com/resources.*

*I like to dip these bad boys in a generous amount of mustard or a 1:1 mix of organic ketchup and mayo. These tend to go great with any meat recipe, particularly steak, salmon, or roast chicken.*

*If you've already experimented with carrots, I recommend trying zucchini or taro for your first batch of tubers.*

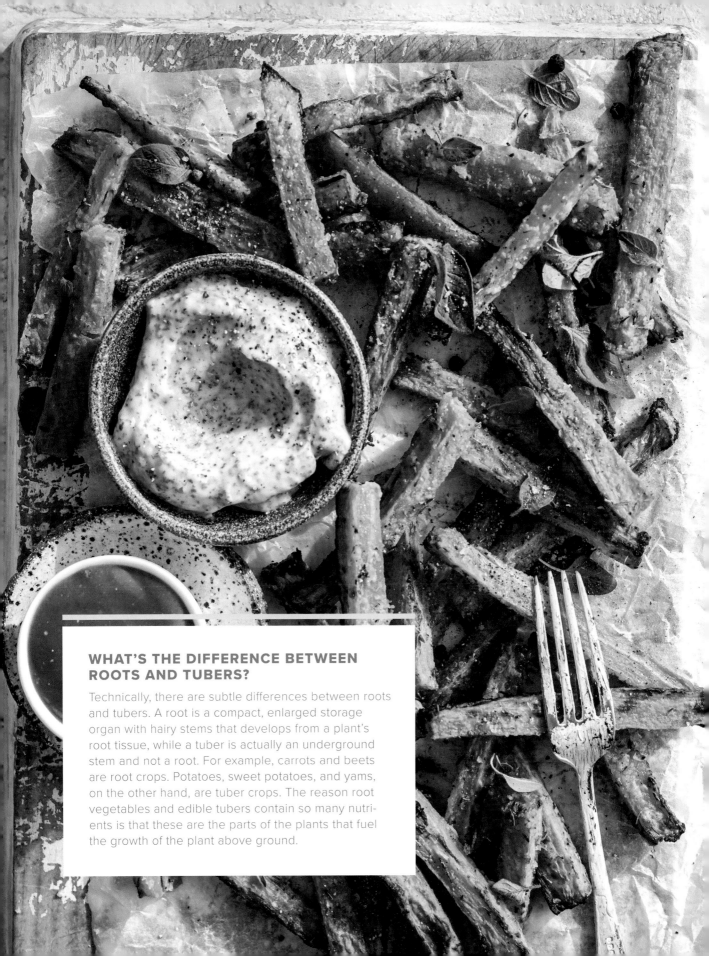

## WHAT'S THE DIFFERENCE BETWEEN ROOTS AND TUBERS?

Technically, there are subtle differences between roots and tubers. A root is a compact, enlarged storage organ with hairy stems that develops from a plant's root tissue, while a tuber is actually an underground stem and not a root. For example, carrots and beets are root crops. Potatoes, sweet potatoes, and yams, on the other hand, are tuber crops. The reason root vegetables and edible tubers contain so many nutrients is that these are the parts of the plants that fuel the growth of the plant above ground.

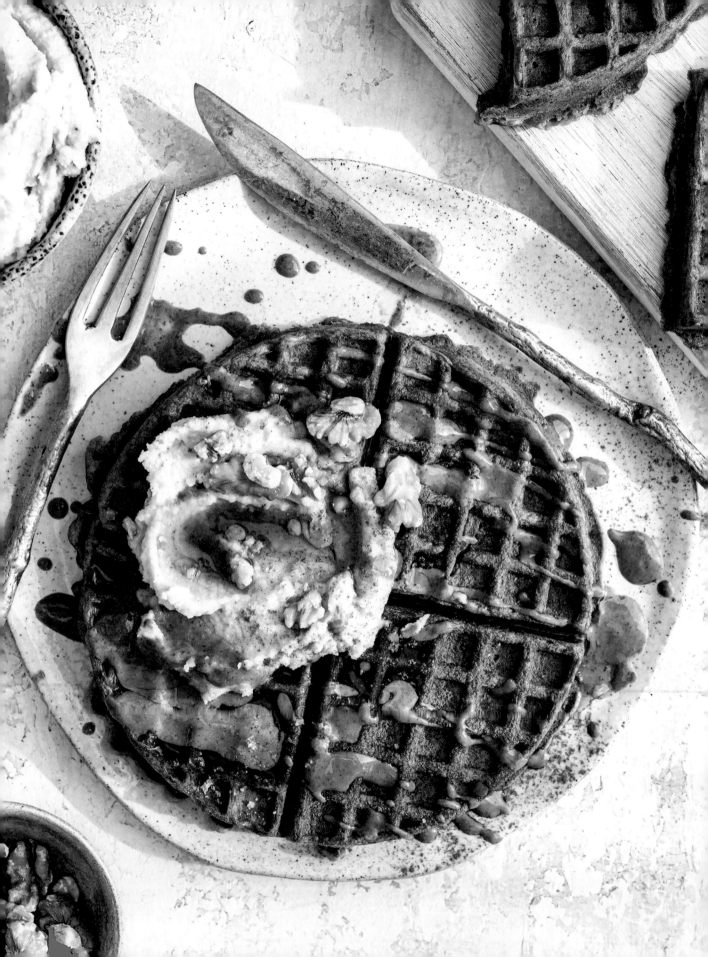

# Carrot Cake Blender Waffles

I'm a sucker for a good waffle. I'm an even bigger sucker for a dense, moist, pinch-me-now-I'm-dreaming carrot cake. So when I ate a carrot cake waffle for the first time, I knew it would be a special dietary staple for the rest of my life. It falls right into the same category as smoked turkey piled with mashed sweet potato and serves as one of the rare highly acceptable substitutions for my usual smoothie breakfast. If you're able to try this recipe with the cashew cream frosting (optional, recipe follows), you may find yourself unable to enjoy a Saturday morning ever again without this magical inclusion.

1. Place all the wet ingredients except the grated carrots in a blender or food processor. Blend for about 30 seconds. Add the flour and blend for another 30 seconds. Add the rest of the dry ingredients and blend until the batter is thick.

2. Add the grated carrots and mix them by hand into the batter. As you mix, heat up a waffle iron, preferably greased with olive oil or avocado oil spray.

3. Scoop out about ½ cup of the batter onto the waffle iron, starting from the middle and moving outward. Close the waffle iron and cook for 4 to 5 minutes, or until the desired crispiness (you know you're getting close when steam disappears).

4. Remove the waffle with a fork.

5. Top with organic maple syrup and almond or walnut butter or—better yet—cashew cream frosting (see recipe below).

*Yield:* 4 SERVINGS

*Total Time:* 30 MINUTES

### TOOLS AND MATERIALS

Blender or food processor

Waffle iron

### WET INGREDIENTS

4 tablespoons melted coconut oil or avocado oil

3 medium or large eggs

1 cup organic goat or cow milk, or a plant-based milk (unsweetened almond or coconut milk works well)

1 teaspoon natural vanilla extract

1 tablespoon apple cider vinegar

¼ cup coconut sugar

1 cup grated carrots

### DRY INGREDIENTS

1 cup gluten-free flour mix (almond flour, coconut flour, Bob's Red Mill, etc.)

¼ cup arrowroot powder, potato starch, or tapioca starch

½ teaspoon salt

2 teaspoon baking powder

1 teaspoon baking soda

1 teaspoon guar gum

1 teaspoon cinnamon

¼ teaspoon ground cloves

¼ teaspoon ground ginger

⅛ teaspoon ground cardamom

# Cashew Cream Waffle Frosting

1. Place the soaked and rinsed cashews, lemon juice, vanilla, powdered sugar, and salt in a blender or food processor.

2. While it mixes, slowly pour in the milk. Then slowly pour in the melted coconut oil and colostrum, if using.

3. Continue to blend or mix until the frosting is smooth (add additional milk 1 tablespoon at a time if necessary to get the mixture silky smooth).

4. Serve immediately on waffles or keep it in the refrigerator for 30 minutes or longer to make it more firm and spreadable.

*Yield:* 4 SERVINGS

*Total Time:* 15 MINUTES, PLUS 3 TO 4 HOURS CASHEW SOAKING TIME (FOR OPTIONAL FROSTING)

## TOOLS AND MATERIALS

Blender or food processor

## INGREDIENTS

2 cups raw cashews soaked for 3 to 4 hours in room-temperature water and then rinsed

2 tablespoons fresh lemon juice

2 teaspoons pure vanilla extract

¾ cup organic powdered sugar, monk fruit, or stevia, to taste

⅛ teaspoon salt

¼ cup coconut milk

¼ cup coconut oil, melted

2 tablespoons colostrum (optional)

**Note:** *Colostrum is optional but highly recommended for added nutty creaminess and gut nourishment. Any leftover waffles can be stored and kept fresh wrapped in parchment paper in the freezer for up to 8 weeks and can be defrosted Eggo-style in a toaster if you'd like.*

## THESE WAFFLES ARE BOTH HEALTHY AND DELICIOUS

This recipe perfectly illustrates why you don't need to go all the way to the far corners of the Orient or the Amazon to hunt down some of the best superfoods. In a recent study that investigated the total antioxidant content of more than 3,100 foods, beverages, spices, herbs, and supplements used worldwide, cloves—the same spice used in this recipe—turned out to be one of the most dense sources of antioxidants in the entire dietary kingdom. Chew on that fact while you chew on these delicious waffles.

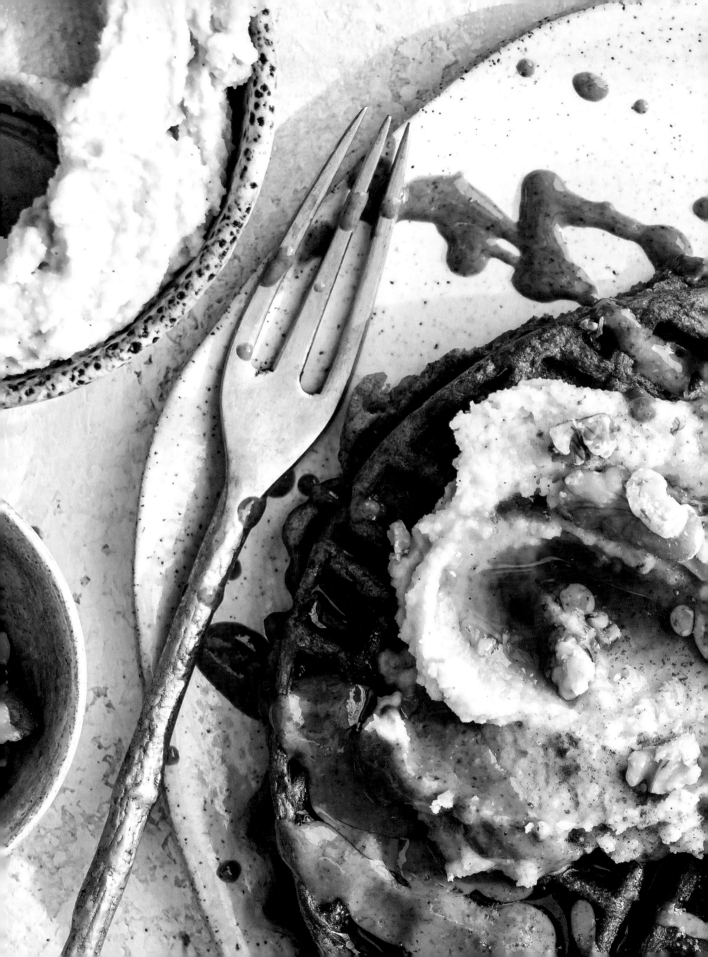

# Parsnip Purée

*Yield:* 4 SERVINGS

*Total Time:* 20 MINUTES

**TOOLS AND MATERIALS**

Blender or food processor

**INGREDIENTS**

1 pound peeled and sliced parsnips

½ cup milk or coconut milk

3 tablespoons ghee or butter, plus more as desired

½ teaspoon salt, plus more to taste

½ teaspoon black pepper, plus more to taste

Butter for serving (optional)

Herbs to taste (optional: dill, paprika, oregano, chives, or garlic)

My wife often whips up this creamy and decadent parsnip purée as a side for dinner. It's versatile and ridiculously easy to prepare, and it serves as a healthy, lower-calorie, lower-carbohydrate alternative to mashed potatoes. I recommend pairing it with any of the meat dishes in this cookbook (heck, I even use it as a "dipping" sauce for my fish, chicken, and steak).

1. Place the peeled and sliced parsnips in a pot and cover them with water. Add a pinch of salt and bring the water to a boil. Boil until the parsnips are fork tender (about 15 minutes) and then drain.

2. Place the drained parsnips in the blender or food processor with the remaining ingredients and blend to a creamy purée. If necessary, add more milk during blending for desired consistency (about that of mashed potatoes or a thick pudding is good).

3. Do a final taste for seasoning, add more salt and pepper if desired, and serve (preferably with a generous dollop of butter!). Just like with mashed potatoes, other herbs and spices can also be fantastic additions.

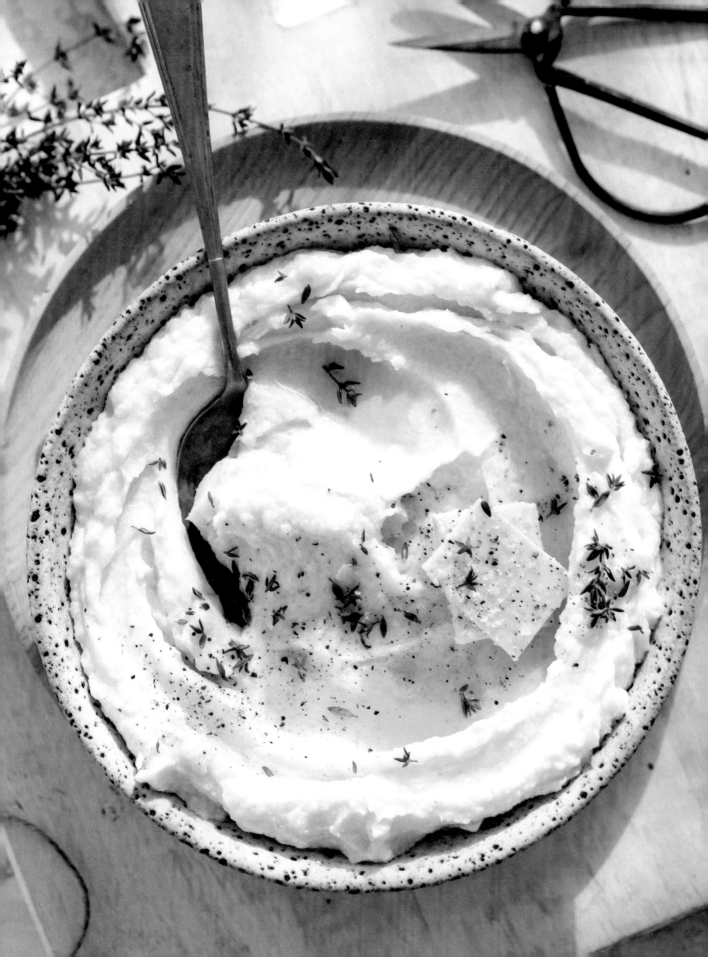

# Meats

Despite what the popular news headlines might have you believe, eating meat is not going to kill you. Unless, that is, you're mowing down on greasy hamburgers and gas station beef jerky and possibly washing it down with that fifth of whiskey and chasing it all with a cigarette. Sure, there *can* be a problem with meat consumption, and the reason meat *could* be bad for you is multifactorial.

*For all resources, books, tools, and ingredients mentioned throughout this chapter, go to: BoundlessKitchen.com/ resources*

First, especially in Western diets, we myopically consume muscle meat. You know: the good ol' ground beef and ribeye steak and dry chicken breast approach. Problem is, muscle meat is quite rich in the amino acid methionine but relatively low in the amino acid glycine. I don't know about you, but I observe most people consuming more of those methionine sources than glycine sources. A high intake of methionine—along with too little glycine—may promote a variety of chronic diseases by causing an imbalance in your body and a buildup of inflammatory compounds such as homocysteine, particularly in people who are genetically susceptible to homocysteine accumulation due to a genetic mutation in a methylation-related gene. Methionine is quite abundant in eggs, seafood, and muscle meat. But glycine is found in high amounts in skin, connective tissue, ligaments, tendons, cartilage, and bones.

Second, when you eat any part of an animal, you're eating and accumulating whatever that animal ate, and that includes any toxins, hormones, and damaged fatty acids. Many animals are fed unhealthy, unnatural food sources and aren't treated or slaughtered humanely; if you're not choosing your meat sources carefully, you probably aren't doing your body (or the planet) many favors. The rise of the modern meat production industry, with its crowded spaces, supplemental hormones, antibiotics, and herbicides and pesticides, has significantly modified not only the quality of conventional meat products but their composition on a molecular level. Research suggests that the protein structures within conventionally produced meat and poultry possess the tendency to become truncated and misfolded into protein structures known as amyloids, which are not destroyed even with a high-temperature cooking process. Over time, our bodies have shown difficulty in the assimilation of these altered protein structures. The heightened presence of amyloids in the body is linked to innumerable chronic diseases, including type 1 diabetes, Alzheimer's, Parkinson's, and autoimmune disease.

Third, certain forms of meat tend to be less nutrient-dense. Thousands of years ago, animal meats were hunted in their natural habitats. They lived and grazed in ample uncrowded spaces. Wild game is the original grass-fed, free-range, sustainable meat source, and naturally raised, grass-fed, grass-finished, pastured animals tend to be leaner, relatively higher in healthy omega-3 fatty acids, and often lower in cholesterol, making their meat a better protein source for people concerned about inflammation and chronic disease. These meats are less tainted by steroids, antibiotics, and other additives, and are also richer in minerals, especially zinc, selenium, and iron due in part to their natural diet as opposed to the grain and corn that are fed to most domesticated animals.

Finally, try to include some wild meat. If you're not a mighty hunter, or friends with one, you can often find wild meat, fish, and fowl selections at most larger grocers. National chains such as Costco, Food Lion, Giant, Harris Teeter, Kroger, and Publix, as well as Trader Joe's and Whole Foods, carry a surprising selection of wild game.

At these mainstream stores, the typical wild animal proteins you will find include buffalo, lamb, bison, Cornish game hen, duck, wild fish, and shellfish. Smaller specialty stores might also include wild boar, pheasant, venison, antelope, elk, and other wild cuts. Your local farmer's market is another perfect place to look. Finally, online providers such as *Wild Idea Buffalo Company*, *Fossil Farms*, and *The Spruce Eats* are other options.

So now that you know I give meat—at least when consumed wisely—a big ol' thumbs up, let's delve into some of my favorite ways to eat it, organs and all.

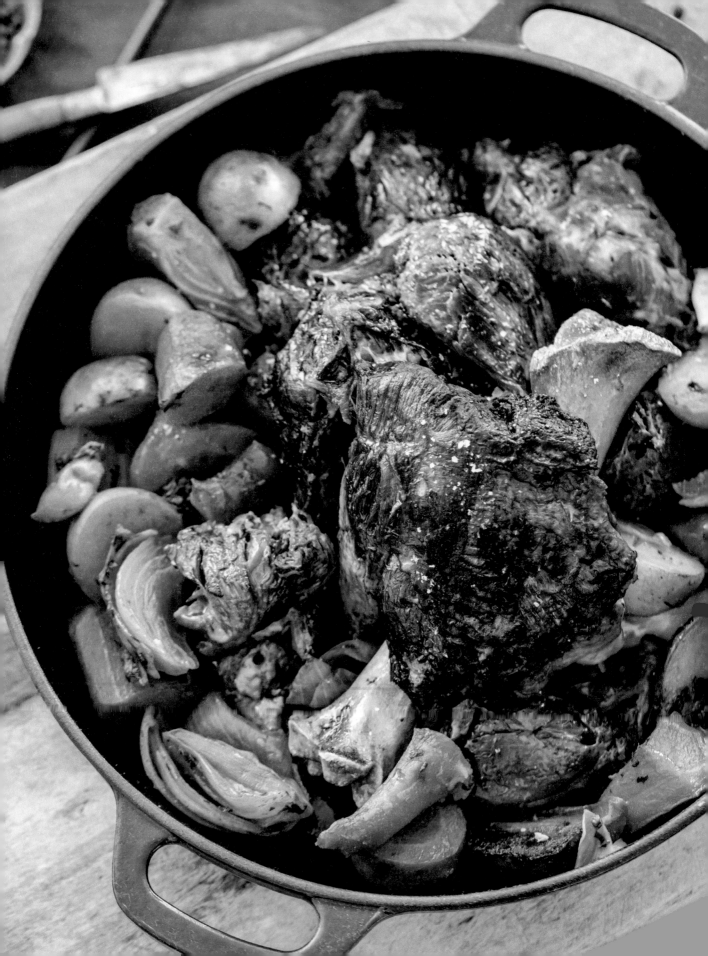

# Wild Game Roast

Ever since I began bowhunting for animals such as whitetail deer, elk, wild boar, goat, sheep, and turkey, I have loved the rugged, natural taste of well-prepared wild game. Not all the game I eat is "wild" per se, but I try to include more than just domesticated animals in my diet, most notably because of wild game's lower concentration of amyloids, which are misfolded protein structures that have been linked to everything from cancer and leaky gut to Alzheimer's.

The following method of preparing wild game is one of those "stupid easy" recipes that will impress your friends and family and make them think you're some crazy fancy French chef, when you're really just mixing up a few ingredients in a roasting pan and walking away. It is a classic "set it and forget it" roasting technique that results in a melt-in-your-mouth taste. It is also perfect for tenderizing the slightly tough or gamy nature of wild meat, such as a cut of venison or leg of mutton—though it will do the trick for just about any cut of meat.

The biggest key for any roast, especially if you find that your roasts seem to come out too chewy, rubbery, dry, or hard, is to cook the roast for a long time at a low temperature. For example, if you're using a slow cooker on meat, you should usually prepare it on low for a good eight to nine hours, or until the meat is falling-apart tender. In an oven set at no higher than 350°F, you'll still want to allow for at least three hours. For that reason, on the days when I want to serve this dish for dinner, I just prepare it all while I'm heating up the water for my morning coffee or tea, and surprisingly, the preparation doesn't take much longer than that. It just comes down to seasoning; acid; a decent roasting liquid like wine, stock, or bone broth; and a few vegetables. The searing step can amplify the flavor and texture even more but is totally optional, and I only sear about half the time.

1. If you're using an oven, preheat it to 300°F (or 350°F, depending on your available cook time).

2. Dry the roast with a paper towel to remove any liquid or blood. Rub 2 tablespoons of the salt all over the meat. You can crosshatch the meat first with a knife if you want the salt to penetrate a bit more deeply.

3. Heat the fat in a large skillet over medium-high heat and sear the roast on all sides until it's lightly browned (this step is optional, but helpful for adding color and flavor to the meat).

4. Remove the roast from the skillet and place it in the bottom of a slow cooker or into a large roasting pan or Dutch oven.

*Yield:* 6 TO 8 SERVINGS

*Total Time:* 20 MINUTES, PLUS UP TO 9 HOURS COOKING TIME

## TOOLS AND MATERIALS

Slow cooker or simply a roasting pan or Dutch oven and an oven

## INGREDIENTS

3- to 4-pound wild game roast

3 tablespoons salt (divided)

1 tablespoon high heat–tolerant cooking fat (such as avocado oil, butter, ghee, or lard)

1½ cups bone broth or chicken stock

1 cup organic red wine

2 tablespoons tomato paste

¼ cup apple cider vinegar

1½ teaspoons Worcestershire sauce

1 teaspoon dried thyme (or a few heaping tablespoons fresh chopped thyme)

1 teaspoon dried parsley (or a few heaping tablespoons of fresh chopped parsley)

1 teaspoon black pepper

5 minced garlic cloves, divided

1 large yellow onion, cut into large pieces

1 pound baby yellow potatoes (optional)

4 to 5 carrots, peeled and sliced into 1- to 2-inch chunks

2 bay leaves

2 tablespoons tapioca starch, arrowroot powder, or cornstarch (optional, for gravy)

**5.** Pour the stock into the bottom of the slow cooker, pan, or Dutch oven. Add the tomato paste, apple cider vinegar, Worcestershire sauce, thyme, parsley, pepper, half the garlic, and 1 tablespoon salt, trying to cover the meat as much as possible with all ingredients.

**6.** Add the onion, potatoes (if using), and carrots on top. Sprinkle on any remaining salt and the remaining garlic.

**7.** Set the slow cooker to low and cook for 8 to 9 hours (or until meat is falling-apart tender). If you're using the oven, cook 3 to 4 hours, or cook for 2 to 3 hours on the higher heat setting. Remember, longer, lower cooking times are best if you have the available time.

**8.** Allow meat to rest and cool for at least 20 minutes before serving. Slice and serve it with the veggies and potatoes and, preferably, an extra mug for all that tasty broth (or make gravy, as instructed below).

**9.** If you opt to make the gravy, whisk the cornstarch, tapioca, or arrowroot powder with about ¼ cup of the strained pot drippings to make a thick slurry. Add the rest of the drippings and the stock to a small saucepan with that slurry and reduce over medium-low heat for 10 minutes, stirring a few times with the whisk as it reduces.

**10.** Enjoy, particularly on a chilly fall or winter evening, with a few slices of sourdough bread for some dipping goodness.

**Note:** *Regarding meat, I'm a big fan of a cut of venison or a giant leg of mutton, but other options include elk, bison, and moose. For a real treat, swap out the apple cider vinegar for any of the artisanal vinegars from my friend T. J. Robinson at GreenfieldPantry .com, which you can learn more about in my podcast with T. J. at bengreenfieldlife.com/ vinegarpodcast.*

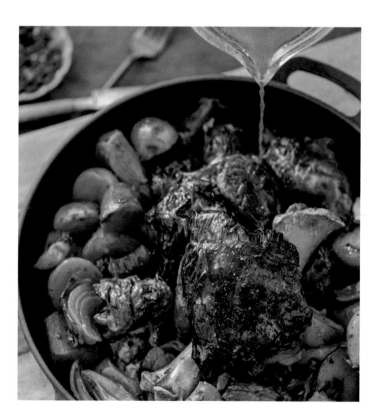

# Tongue Tacos (Tacos de Lengua)

Yes, I know eating organ meat (also called "offal") sounds gross or, well, awful. But organ meats can be prepared in amazingly flavorful ways. And when you think about it, there's an ethical and environmental argument for eating an entire animal "nose-to-tail" rather than wasting the majority of an animal (the organs, bones, skin, and other miscellaneous parts) to simply eat the muscle meat.

I personally consume some type of offal three to five times a week, and one of those occasions includes our regularly scheduled "tongue taco" night at the Greenfield house.

Beef tongue is well known for its unique taste. The blast of flavor partially comes from beef tongue's high fat content. Because of this fat content, tongue also contains various fatty acids that mix together into a tender texture and a mild but pleasant taste. Tongue also contains a host of B vitamins and is particularly rich in vitamin $B_{12}$, which helps support healthy brain and nerve function by insulating nerves and keeping blood cells healthy. While $B_{12}$ helps nerve function, choline—another significant component of tongue—assists significantly with nerve communication. Finally, tongue is quite high in iron and zinc, assisting with production of hemoglobin (a protein that supplies oxygen to your body) and wound healing, fighting infections, and immune system function.

Here's my favorite method for consuming organ meat: the mighty tongue taco, which is such a hit for anyone lucky enough to join my family for tongue taco night that I'm frequently told it's the best taco filling ever—superior to fish, beef, chicken, or any other common taco protein. Warning: after consuming, you may find yourself signing and/or speaking Spanish with greater fluency the next day. Or perhaps that's just a placebo effect.

**1.** Place the tongue in your pot of choice. I recommend a slow cooker for this recipe, but you can also fill any large stock pot with water (or bone broth) to cover. Add onions, crushed garlic cloves, bay leaves, peppercorns, and salt.

**2.** Set the slow cooker on low for 7 to 8 hours, or if you're using a regular stock pot, bring the water to a boil, reduce the heat to a simmer, cover, and cook tongue on low heat for 3 to 4 hours, until the tongue is soft to the touch and tender.

**3.** Remove the tongue from the water and let it cool for 5 minutes. Then, using your fingers or a sharp small knife, remove the thin, skin-like covering of the tongue and discard it (or feed it to your hungry feline or canine friends).

*Yield:* 4 SERVINGS

*Total Time:* 4 TO 8 HOURS

## TOOLS AND MATERIALS

Slow cooker or simply a large stock pot

## INGREDIENTS

1 3- to 4-pound beef tongue

2 large onions, peeled

1 entire head of garlic cloves, peeled and crushed

6 to 7 bay leaves

1 tablespoon peppercorns

2 tablespoons salt

2 large pats (about 2 tablespoons) butter

8 Tortillas

2 avocados, chopped

1 red onion, chopped

1 large bunch cilantro, chopped

½ cup thinly sliced radishes for garnish (I of course recommend using the Quick Pickled Onions or Radishes on page 71!)

Salsa and/or hot sauce

Sour cream or plain full-fat yogurt (optional)

***Note:*** *Tongue is easy to find at local Asian markets, Mexican markets, or at your local butcher, although I order mine from US Wellness Meats. For tortillas, I recommend Siete brand, which makes an assortment of grain-free tortilla and tortilla hard shells, including almond, cassava, and chickpea. For salsas I like Thrive Market or your own homemade salsa, and for hot sauce, Joey's Organic Hot Sauce.*

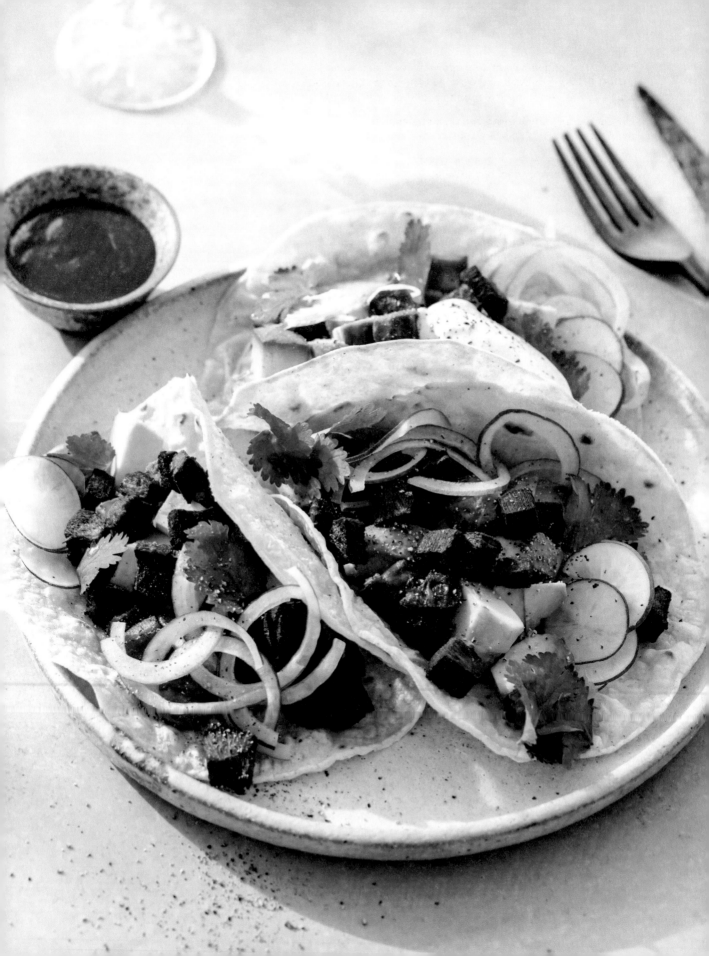

**4.** Cube the tongue by cutting it into strips and then cutting each strip into somewhat equal-size ¼-inch pieces (if you like, you can sauté the strips first and then cut them into cubes).

**5.** Heat the butter in a frying pan on medium-high heat and sauté the cubes until they are lightly browned.

**6.** While you are frying the tongue, or after, crisp up the tortillas by lightly frying them on the stove top until pockets of air appear in them.

**7.** Make your tacos! Place a large spoonful of cubed tongue in the center of a tortilla. Add a spoonful of salsa and a generous helping of avocado, onion, and cilantro. Garnish with the radish slices, along with hot sauce, salt, and pepper to taste. Some folks, like me, also enjoy a giant dollop of sour cream or yogurt.

## HEALTH BENEFITS OF ORGAN MEAT

The health benefits of organ meats are the most compelling reason to consume these odd bits. There are two important considerations here:

1. **More glycine:** Most modern protein consumers, due to a diet shifted in an unbalanced manner toward primarily muscle meat consumption, are eating tons of *methionine* and barely any *glycine*. Why is this a problem? Studies show that methionine restriction can increase lifespan and improve most factors of metabolic health, such as body fat, insulin sensitivity, blood lipids, and liver health. But getting more glycine into the diet can help balance out these excess methionine levels.

2. **High nutrient density:** organ meats are truly "nature's multivitamin," with a much higher nutrient density than common so-called "superfoods" such as kale, blueberries, spirulina, or any other fancy overpriced fad plant. Organ meats are particularly good sources of B vitamins, such as vitamin $B_{12}$ and folate. They are packed full of minerals, including magnesium, iron, zinc, and selenium. And they also contain important fat-soluble vitamins like vitamins A, D, E, and K.

Finally, should you be concerned about the myth that organ meats such as kidneys and liver are "filters" filled with toxins: don't be. These organs don't filter toxins by trapping them in tissue and keeping them there; rather, they shunt them out into urine and feces, where they quickly exit the body. So unless you're eating an animal's bladder and colon, you'll be just fine (as with all meat, I recommend you buy your organ meats from clean, grass-fed, grass-finished sources).

# Ben's Biohacked, Braised, and Boundless Beef Stew

Bourguignon (pronounced "boor-geen-yuhn") is a traditional French beef stew braised in red wine and beef stock, typically flavored with carrots, onions, garlic, and select herbs and spices and garnished with pearl onions, mushrooms, and bacon.

My own twist on bourguignon is a "biohacked" (hey, I had to add in an extra "b"!) method that really amplifies the flavor of just about any stew meat, roast meat, or even organ meat, if you decide to use that. It's actually a fast and easy way to feed yourself or a whole family for days, since most stews taste even better in the days after cooking.

Braising the meat with elements like maple syrup and vinegar gives the fibers plenty of time to become fall-apart tender while all the flavor sinks deep into the ingredients. As a bonus, the braising liquid reduces to a thick, concentrated sauce to pour over the meat on your plate and add extra flavor to the caramelized vegetables included in this recipe as well. The optional red juice powder is a fantastic way to add extra caramelization and nutrients to this recipe.

For an incredibly even cook with no "hot spots" and a nice outdoor cooking experience, I like to cook this one in my Dutch oven on my Traeger grill, although an oven works just fine.

## BEEF PREPARATION INSTRUCTIONS

1. Preheat your oven or grill to 350°F.

2. In a large bowl, combine the broth, wine, apple cider vinegar, maple syrup, and hot sauce and/or tomato paste.

3. Over low to medium heat on the stovetop, in the Dutch oven, melt the butter (for about 2 minutes). Add the bacon and sizzle for about 8 to 10 minutes, until lightly browned.

4. Add the meat, onions, and garlic. Brown the meat evenly on all sides, which will take about another 5 to 6 minutes. To brown the meat evenly, you may need to add it in separate batches.

5. Add the gluten-free flour, sea salt, black pepper, and Organifi Red powder (if using), and stir all the powder ingredients together until no dry ingredients are visible and the meat is evenly coated.

6. Pour the liquid ingredients in the bowl over the top of the meat and stir thoroughly until all ingredients are mixed together.

7. Place the Dutch oven in the oven or on the grill and cook for 2 hours and 30 minutes.

---

*Yield:* 6 TO 8 SERVINGS

*Total Time:* 3 HOURS

**TOOLS AND MATERIALS:**

Oven or grill

Dutch oven

**INGREDIENTS FOR THE BEEF**

2 cups organic bone broth

1 cup organic biodynamic wine

⅔ cup apple cider vinegar

⅔ cup organic maple syrup

1 tablespoon Joey's Hot Sauce and/or 1 tablespoon tomato paste

4 tablespoons Kerrygold butter or any other grass-fed, grass-finished butter

10 to 12 slabs of bacon, cut into small rectangular pieces with scissors or knife

5 pounds chuck roast or stew meat, chopped into approximately 1-inch chunks

1 red or white onion, minced

3 garlic cloves, minced

½ cup gluten-free flour or Himalayan tartary buckwheat flour

Salt and black pepper, to taste

2 heaping scoops Organifi Red Juice powder (optional)

1 tablespoon organic herbes de Provence seasoning (a mixture of dried herbs typically consisting of savory, rosemary, basil, thyme, and oregano)

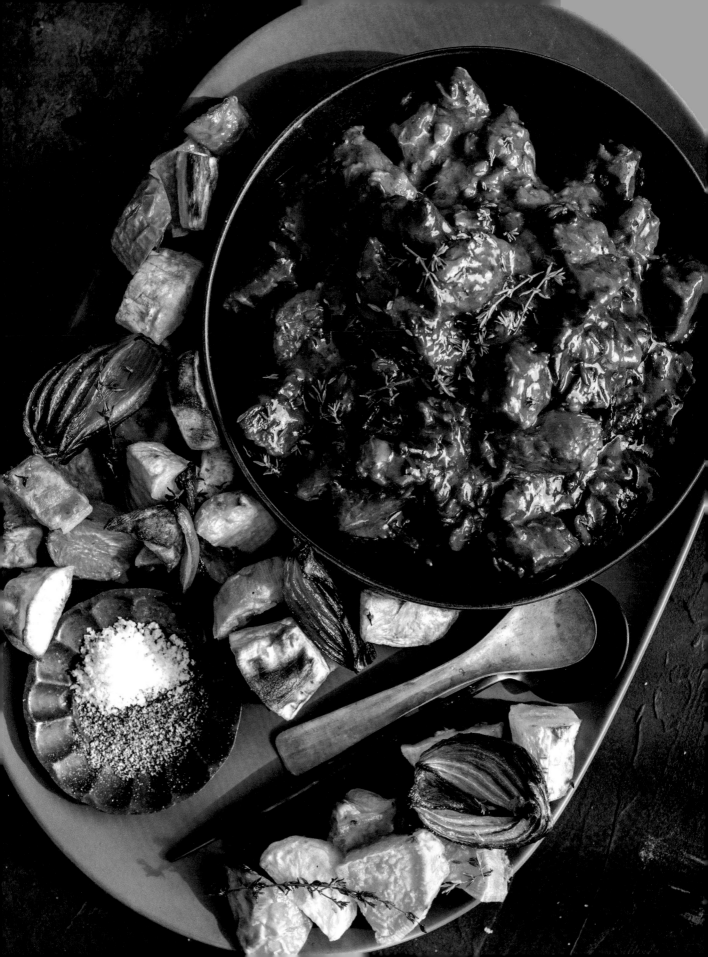

## VEGETABLE PREPARATION INSTRUCTIONS

**1.** Preheat the oven to 350°F.

**2.** In a bowl, combine the carrots, potatoes, parsnips, red onion, garlic cloves, olive oil, and honey (maple syrup) if using. Season to taste with Colima salt and black pepper.

**3.** Spread the vegetables out over a baking sheet or casserole dish, top with the sprig of fresh thyme, and cook in the preheated oven or on the grill for 30 to 40 minutes.

**4.** If you are eating right away, simply plate the caramelized vegetables and spoon the meat and sauce over them.

One tasty twist on this recipe is to simply throw all the vegetable ingredients into the Dutch oven along with the meat and cook everything together, although your vegetables will be less caramelized and crunchy if you do this.

Finally, it should go without saying that serving the stew with a slice of my wife's world-famous sourdough bread recipe (for slathering in the sauce) is an absolute slice of heaven.

## INGREDIENTS FOR THE VEGETABLES

4 carrots, chopped

2 sweet potatoes, peeled and diced

3 parsnips, peeled and sliced

1 red onion, quartered

2 garlic cloves, minced

½ cup extra virgin olive oil

2 tablespoons organic maple syrup or honey (optional)

Colima salt and freshly ground black pepper

1 sprig fresh thyme

***Note:*** *In addition to chuck roast or stew meat, I have also experimented successfully with using heart or liver that has been soaked in buttermilk or kefir for 24 hours and then rinsed and chopped. There's just something about sitting in this stew for a few hours that makes organ meats delicious. Regarding timing, if you plan to eat the meat right away, just slip the vegetables into the same oven or grill as the meat at close to the 2-hour mark of the meat cooking. This recipe is absolutely fantastic the next day or two days later as well, so you can also pop it into the fridge and save it for later or have leftovers the next day!*

## A MAKE-IT-YOUR-WAY BOURGUIGNON

Admittedly, one of my goals with this stew was to creatively use the variety of unique ingredients I had found scattered about my pantry—a strategy possibly considered by some real chefs to be a bastardization of a traditional French bourguignon but, in my opinion, a significant and very nutrient-dense health upgrade. Specifically, I included grass-fed, grass-finished beef, and pastured bacon from US Wellness Meats; Kettle & Fire organic bone broth; the antioxidant-rich Organifi Red Juice powder; a touch of organic Joey's Hot Sauce; the incredible, antioxidant-rich Angelica Mill Himalayan tartary buckwheat flour; organic, biodynamic wine from Dry Farm Wines; Fresh-Pressed Olive Oil Club extra virgin olive oil; and a bit of the incredibly flavorful Colima salt from the Mexican coast.

# Sous Vide Pork Belly *with* Vinegar Deglaze Sauce

Pork belly definitely qualifies as one of my happy foods, but sous vide pork belly is sure to plaster a giant, satisfied smile on your face. Using the sous vide technique (see page 45) allows you to create a perfectly juicy and tender belly every single time, along with a joyful crispy exterior crunch when you finish the sous vide pork belly with a final sear. I've discovered that the sweet spot temperature and time for a perfectly tender and juicy pork belly is a 165°F sous vide water bath for 10 hours, followed by a final sear, either in a pan, with a blow torch, in an air fryer, or under a broiler.

While the "deglaze" step is optional, it's worth learning how to do it so you can make incredible sauces that pair perfectly with any meat, poultry, fish, or vegetable dish. Deglazing is actually quite simple and is done by adding a small amount of vinegar (or sometimes wine or beer) to the pan you've cooked the meat in. Then you stir to loosen the browned bits of protein and fat on the bottom of the pan, which are technically referred to in the culinary sciences as the *fond*—a fancy French word which I'm guessing means "very flavorful brown sludgy particles."

The deglaze mixture can then be transformed into a tasty sauce to accompany any food cooked in the pan. A side bonus of deglazing is that it makes cleaning up the pan afterward a much faster and easier process.

## INSTRUCTIONS FOR THE PORK BELLY

1. Generously salt and pepper all sides of the pork belly.

2. Set a sous vide wand to 165°F.

3. Place the pork in a sous vide bag, and make sure there's no air in the bag. Drop the bag into a sous vide bath in a large stock pot and let the pork belly cook for 10 hours.

4. Remove the pork belly from sous vide bag and dry it with paper towels. Transfer it to an oiled pan on the stove top.

5. Sear the pork belly fat side down at medium-high temperature for 1 to 2 minutes per side, or until crispy (use this method if you plan to deglaze). For this step you could also air fry it for 5 to 6 minutes, sear it with a blowtorch until all sides of the pork belly are crispy, or place it under the broiler in the oven for 2 to 3 minutes.

6. Place the seared pork belly on a plate to rest for 5 minutes.

*Yield:* 4 TO 6 SERVINGS

*Total Time:* 10 HOURS

## TOOLS AND MATERIALS

Sous vide wand and sous vide bags

Large stock pot for sous vide

Pan for deglaze/pork belly sear process

Air fryer, blowtorch (optional)

## INGREDIENTS

1 to 2 pounds pork belly, skin removed

Salt, to taste

Black pepper, to taste

Oil for pan

Red onions (optional)

Butter

A few tablespoons vinegar, wine, or beer (optional, for the deglaze)

1 tablespoon butter or heavy cream (optional, for the deglaze)

**Note:** *For this dish, I recommend any of T. J. Robinson's artisanal vinegars, from GreenfieldPantry .com. If I'm not deglazing, I prefer to air fry.*

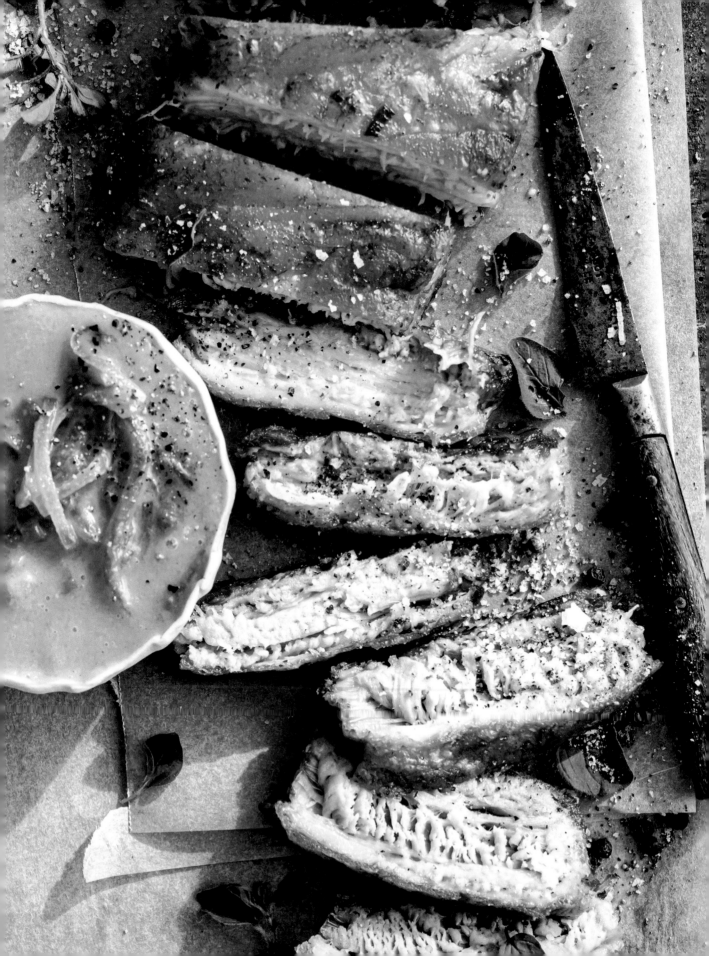

7. Meanwhile, sauté the red onions, if using, in butter to caramelize them, about 10 minutes.

8. Cut the meat into slices, add on onions (if using), drizzle with deglazed vinegar sauce (optional, see below), slice, serve, and enjoy!

### INSTRUCTIONS FOR THE DEGLAZE

1. After you remove the meat from the pan, slightly lower the temperature of the stove top to medium.

2. Pour enough vinegar into the pan to cover any brown bits left in the bottom. You should only need a few tablespoons, just enough to cover the pan by about half an inch. You can use wine or beer if you don't have vinegar.

3. As the liquid heats, scrape the bottom of the pan with a wooden spoon or a plastic or rubber spatula until all the thick "fond" particles are blended in with the liquid. Don't use metal for this as it can damage your pan and sometimes even expose you to toxins and metals that get scraped off the pan.

4. Boil the liquid until it is reduced by half (should only take 4 to 6 minutes) to concentrate the flavor and thicken your sauce. Remove from the heat, whisk in a tablespoon of butter or heavy cream, if using, and serve.

## DEGLAZING DEMYSTIFIED

I first learned about deglazing when I interviewed "Vinegar Hunter" T. J. Robinson on a podcast about all-things-vinegar (bengreenfieldlife.com/vinegarpodcast) and began to receive special shipments of artisanal vinegars from around the world as a part of T. J.'s special vinegar delivery service at GreenfieldPantry.com. Incidentally, that same podcast is where I got the idea to begin maker vinegar-infused shrub cocktails, like those featured on page 89.

# Sous Vide Blueberry Brisket

A properly prepared brisket is widely considered to be the holy grail of the barbecue kingdom. Problem is, it's also easy to mess up brisket and get a disappointingly dry or rubbery result. This is because a lean cut of brisket, with less connective tissue and fat to keep it moist as it cooks, can be tough and leathery if not cooked properly. Traditionally, a long barbecue at a low temperature—including tending to the brisket overnight with a spray bottle and plenty of tender, loving care—was pretty much the only way to get a melt-in-your-mouth, tender brisket.

But now there's another way. Enter sous vide. Sous vide cooking can allow a total barbecue novice to produce a moist and tender brisket that will impress even a Texan. I was blown away when I first tried this recipe, and a multitude of my dinner guests commented that it was the most juicy, succulent, and moist brisket they'd ever experienced.

Yes, yes, I know that sous vide might be a far cry from the rustic, smoky nature of a true barbecue, and may not have quite the complexity or so-called "terroir" of a brisket that's been tended all through the night by a patient and determined pitmaster armed with a flashlight and spritzer bottle. But bear with me here: the texture and ease of the sous vide process, paired with the unparalleled moistness and tenderness you'll enjoy from this recipe, make it worth at least trying. In other words, don't knock sous vide brisket until you've tried it. Plus it's simple: rub the meat down, drop it in the bag, walk away, and then do a quick finish on the grill or in the oven to polish it off.

Temperature and timing vary for this recipe, depending on how much time you have and your ultimate goals for the final brisket texture. If you want the best sous vide brisket experience, I recommend setting the water temperature at 135°F for 40 to 60 hours. If you don't quite have that much time, then 155°F at 30 to 40 hours works and will still give you the tenderness of a medium-rare steak. However, in my opinion, it is nowhere near as good as cooking at the lower temperature for a longer period of time. Any temperatures lower than 135°F or higher than 155°F are basically either too cool to break down muscle fibers to the point that they shred like traditional brisket or too hot, resulting in a dry and leathery meat.

Of course, unless you decide to add a little liquid smoke to your sous vide bag, which is one option, you'll miss out on the traditional smoky barbecue flavor of brisket when using a sous vide method. However, if you own a smoker (ideal), or even just a barbecue grill, you can finish off this recipe with a final cook at 250 to 300°F for two to three additional hours. This will not only give your brisket a traditional smoky flavor but also a crunchy, caramelized crunch.

Finally, dropping a few blueberries into the bag offers a fantastic addition to this recipe. Why? It turns out that an impressive study recently demonstrated that combining a nutrient found in

*Yield:* 8 TO 10 SERVINGS

*Total Time:* 30 TO 60 HOURS

## TOOLS AND MATERIALS

Large stock pot for the sous vide bath

Plastic FoodSaver bags or silicone Stasher bags

Sous vide wand

Vacuum sealer (if using FoodSaver bags)

## INGREDIENTS

1 5- to 10-pound brisket

Approximately ½ cup coarse salt (such as kosher salt)

Approximately ½ cup black pepper

Approximately 1 cup organic blueberries or other desired spices and herbs (optional)

Barbecue sauce (optional)

Salt and black pepper, to taste (if using blueberries, to make sauce)

Butter or extra virgin olive oil (if using blueberries, to make sauce)

***Notes:*** *Breville Joule is a good wand, or you can go for a fancier sous vide setup—Anova and Breville are good. See the Resources section on page 143 for more on sous vide equipment recommendations. For barbecue sauce, you can't go wrong with Primal Kitchen Golden BBQ Sauce.*

*This dish will pair fantastically with not only the buttered-up blueberries, mentioned above, but also with Air-Fried Pickles (see page 19) and Quick Pickled Onions or Radishes (see page 71), along with toasted sourdough bread from the original Boundless Cookbook.*

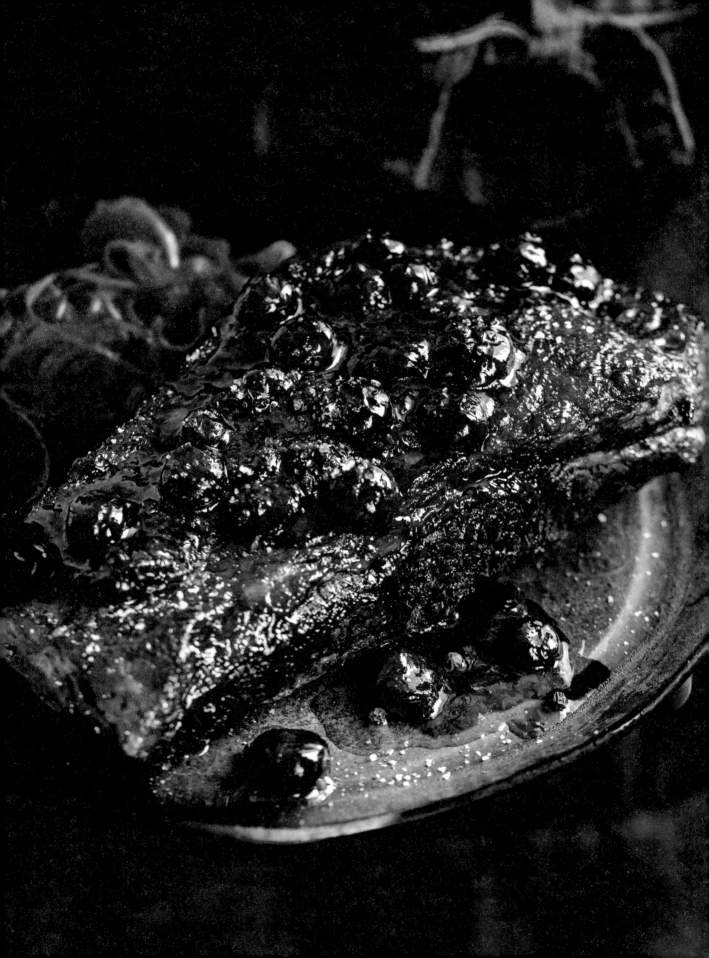

beef (carnosine) with blueberries can send your energy levels skyrocketing. It does this by supercharging your stem cell proliferation by more than 80 percent! The added bonus is that the sweet tartness of the blueberries pairs amazingly with the rich, salty flavor of sous vide beef.

1. Crosshatch the brisket with a knife and then rub salt and pepper evenly over the entire surface.

2. Place the brisket in a FoodSaver-style vacuum bag or a large Stasher bag, or cut it in half across the midsection and put each half into medium Stasher bags. Throw in all the blueberries or any other herbs and spices you desire, if using, and seal the bag completely airtight.

3. Set the sous vide wand to your desired temperature (135 to 155°F) and cook for 30 to 40 hours at 155°F or 40 to 60 hours at 135°F. At this point, you can drench the meat in barbecue sauce and proceed to rest the brisket before serving, or move on to the next step (saving the saucing for later is recommended).

4. If you prefer to finish the brisket with some smoky flavor, allow it to cool to room temperature (about 1 hour) before an oven or smoker process. (To speed up cooling, you can place the brisket bags in an ice bath for 15 minutes or in the refrigerator for an hour and a half.)

5. Remove the brisket from the bag or bags and pat dry, saving the blueberries (if using) for later to make a sauce. Throw them in a pan and stir them up with salt and pepper to taste and the butter, if using. You can serve this as a side sauce or spooned atop the final recipe.

6. Preheat the oven to 250 to 300°F. Finish the brisket in the oven or, preferably, on a smoker, fat cap down, at 250 to 300°F for 2 to 3 hours. If you have a favorite barbeque sauce, you can brush it over the brisket prior to this step.

7. Pull the meat from the heat, and allow to rest for 30 to 60 minutes before slicing it against the grain to the desired thickness and serving. I prefer to wrap the brisket in a bath towel and then place it in a cooler for the entire resting process. This helps the meat maintain its heat for longer by slowing down the cooling process, which means the brisket can stay at a safe temperature for longer before you cut into it.

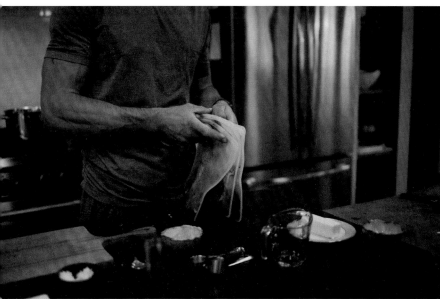
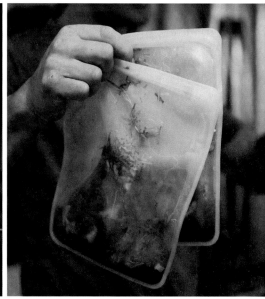

## WHAT IS SOUS VIDE?

Sous vide cooking is simply the process of sealing food in an airtight container—usually a sealed bag—and then cooking that food in temperature-controlled water. Professional chefs use this tactic to get a consistent temperature and texture on meat by vacuum sealing a protein with components such as a marinade of choice oils and vinegars, sauce, herbs, or spices and then dropping the vacuum-sealed protein in a large pot of water. To really see what I mean, and to understand the enormous versatility of the sous vide technique, check out *Sous Vide Everything*, a YouTube channel that's just as entertaining as it sounds.

A sous vide machine typically uses a heated metal coil to warm water to a constant temperature that doesn't fluctuate to high or low extremes. This means that the cooking progress is gradual and controlled. Since the water never goes past the desired temperature of doneness, a sous vide recipe can take a bit longer to cook (a proper sous vide steak can take a couple of hours, compared to just minutes on a grill). But this also means that you'll never have an overcooked piece of protein, and there's really not a lot of actual maintenance required during the cooking process: you just put your chosen meat, marinade, herbs, and spices into a bag, drop the bag into water, set a timer, and walk away. Although there are very fancy and expensive restaurant-grade sous vide setups, I personally use a simple and inexpensive Breville Joule brand sous vide wand, which syncs to my phone and can even send me an alert when my recipe is ready, which is quite convenient. Using the Breville Joule, the only other tools and materials I need are a giant stock pot of water and a good sous vide bag (see below and the Resources section on page 143 for more).

One common concern about sous vide is the potential for plastic leaching into the food. For this reason, I primarily use heat-resistant silicone Stasher bags. This brand is not only better for the planet (you can reuse Stashers over and over again, unlike single-use plastics such as the commonly used FoodSaver bags or Ziplocs, which I only use with a very large cut of meat such as brisket) but, importantly, each bag is made of pure platinum food-grade silicone that is much safer to cook in if you are concerned about unhealthy plastics in your food. With a large Stasher bag, you can sous vide multiple steaks at a time, although I recommend just one steak per bag, especially if you want to experiment with different flavor combinations for each steak, which can make for a fun cooking experience.

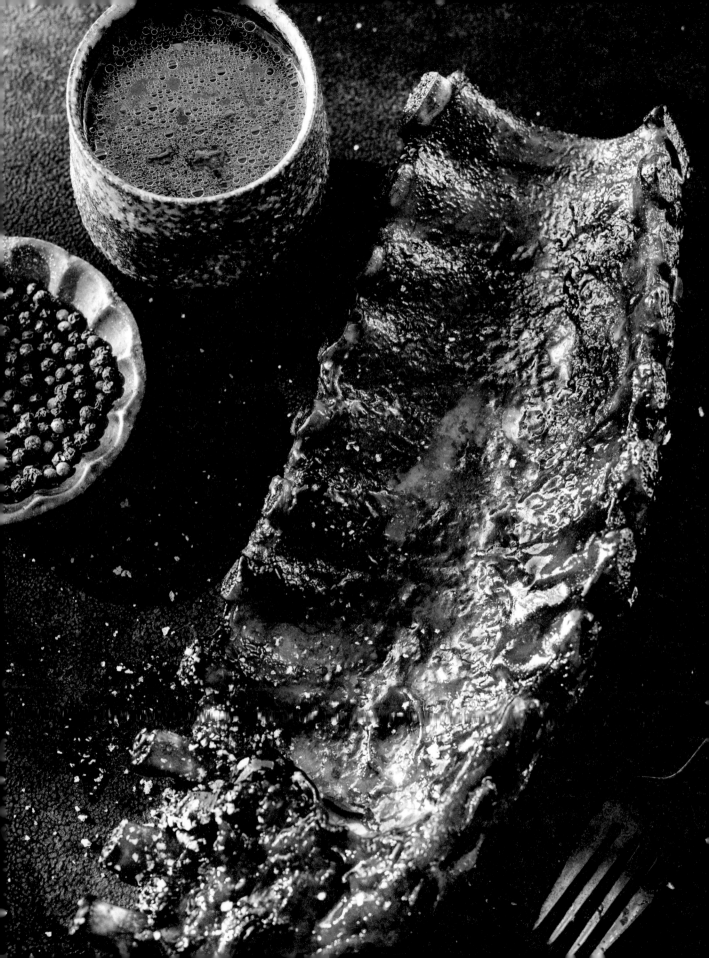

# Time-Hacked Baby Back Ribs

*Yield:* 4 TO 6 SERVINGS

*Total Time:* 50 MINUTES

**TOOLS AND MATERIALS**

Pressure cooker

Large roasting pan

**INGREDIENTS**

½-pound rack of ribs (pork or beef both work)

Per ½ pound rack of ribs:

    1 teaspoon turmeric powder

    1 teaspoon salt

    1 teaspoon black pepper

    ½ teaspoon Ceylon cinnamon

    1 cup organic bone broth

    ½ cup organic red wine

    Barbecue sauce of your choice

*__Note:__ You can use the leftover broth, wine, and spice-infused liquid in the pressure cooker as a flavorful, nutrient-dense beverage to sip from a mug with dinner; or reduce down the liquid into a gravy on the stove top using flour or non-GMO corn starch.*

This unique recipe is an easy way to create melt-in-your-mouth, fall-off-the-bone, tender ribs in just a fraction of the usual cooking time. Your secret weapon for this recipe is a pressure cooker, which works on a simple but very convenient principle: steam pressure. To pressure cook, you put all your ingredients into a sealed pot and then steam inside builds up high pressure, which helps food cook surprisingly faster (in this case, ribs that would normally take me four to six hours of tending on a grill can be completely cooked and ready to eat in under an hour).

Mechanically speaking, a pressure cooker is just a sealed pot with a valve that controls the steam pressure inside. As the pot heats up, the liquid inside forms steam, which raises the pressure in the pot. This high-pressure steam raises the boiling point of the water in the pot and also helps force liquid and moisture into the food, which helps tough meat like ribs get very tender, very quickly. As an added bonus, the flavors created in a pressure cooker can be far more deep and complex compared to regular steaming results. When I found myself short on time and first used this technique on a big rack of baby back beef ribs— followed by a quick, five-minute caramelizing broil after removing the ribs from the pressure cooker—I was quite pleased to realize that I would no longer need to spend hours upon hours tending ribs on the grill.

Please thoroughly read the instructions that accompany your pressure cooker. There are a few subtle nuances you'll want to pay attention to, such as the amount of liquid in the pot, along with the proper buttons and valves to press for pressurizing/ depressurizing. Trust me: you don't want to blow a pressure cooker lid through your kitchen ceiling and spew scalding hot cooking liquids all over the counter.

1. Trim the silver skin off the back of the ribs (optional, but you'll get better texture/cooking if you do this).

2. Rub the ribs thoroughly with the turmeric, salt, black pepper, and Ceylon cinnamon.

3. Place the ribs in the pressure cooker. If you have multiple cuts of ribs, you can layer or stack them.

4. Add the bone broth and red wine to the pressure cooker.

5. Place the lid on the pressure cooker, pressurize, and cook for 30 minutes.

6. Allow the pressure cooker to completely depressurize and then remove the ribs. Finish off by placing the ribs in a roasting pan and drenching generously with barbecue sauce, then broiling in the oven for 5 to 8 minutes to get perfect caramelization.

# Bacon-Wrapped Berry Beef Loin Roast

I recently prepared this beautiful, juicy, bacon-wrapped beef loin roast for my dear mother's birthday, using one of my go-to meat rubs: a superfood berry blend from my original *Boundless Cookbook*. One of my favorite meat rub ingredients of all time for this method happens to be Organifi red juice powder (see Resources on page 143 for more info).

Using this blend of superfoods and blood-building compounds—originally designed to make juices and smoothies—"off-label" as a rub caramelizes and amplifies the flavor of meat in a unique way, while its built-in antioxidants neutralize many of the free radicals and barbecue carcinogens.

1. Lay the loin out on a rack or counter, dry completely with a paper towel, crosshatch with a sharp knife, and rub down thoroughly with your rub of choice.

2. Layer all the slices of bacon on top of the loin.

3. Smoke in a smoker grill at 165°F for 2 hours (optional but recommended); if you skip this step, go straight to roasting or grilling the meat.

4. Preheat the oven to 375°F.

5. Roast in the oven or finish on the grill at 375°F for 40 to 45 minutes (use a meat thermometer and remove the roast from the heat at 135°F for a perfect medium-rare).

6. Let the tenderloin cool and rest for 20 minutes. Slice it into 1/4- to 1/2-inch-thick portions that include both a bit of bacon and a bit of loin and serve with your favorite barbecue sauce.

*Yield:* 6 TO 8 SERVINGS

*Total Time:* 3 HOURS

## TOOLS AND MATERIALS

Oven or barbecue grill and/or smoker

Meat thermometer

## INGREDIENTS

One 4-pound beef tenderloin (about a 1:4 bacon-to-loin ratio)

Rub

*Option 1:* Organifi Red Juice powder

*Option 2:* Pulverize 1 cup dried or dehydrated organic berries of your choice (such as blueberries, cranberries, goji berries, or raspberries) in a blender until finely powdered. Then mix with salt, cinnamon, paprika, and cayenne to desired flavor.

1 pound sliced bacon

Barbecue sauce of your choice

**Note:** *Layering the bacon on top of the loin creates fat that drips down into the meat and lends a fantastic umami flavor to the dish (this is a great tip for any long smoke or BBQ process with a meat that you want to keep moist and juicy).*

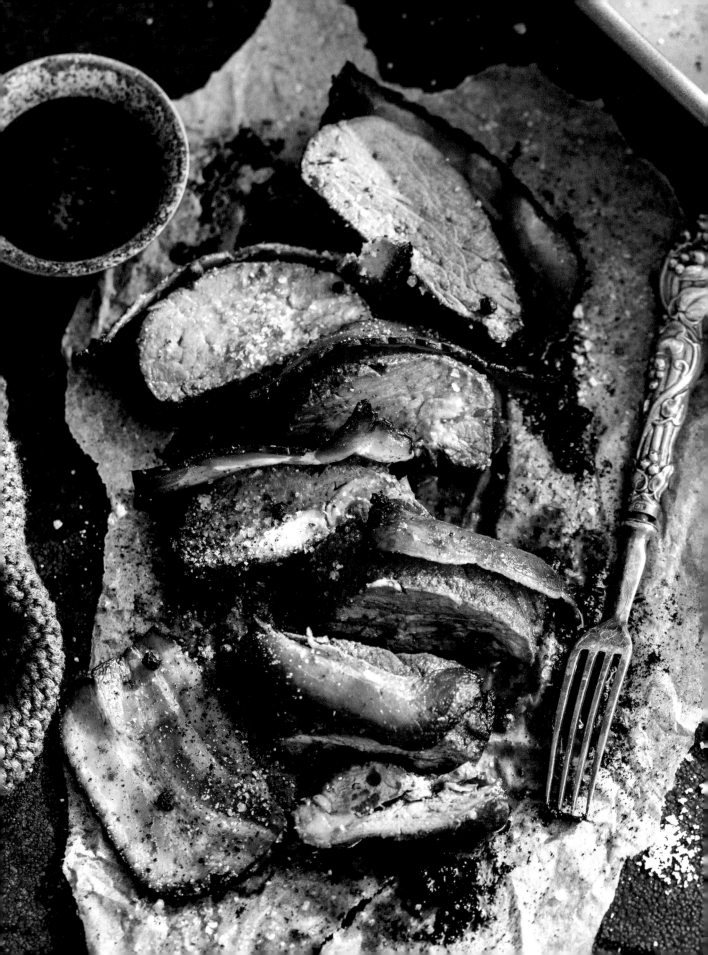

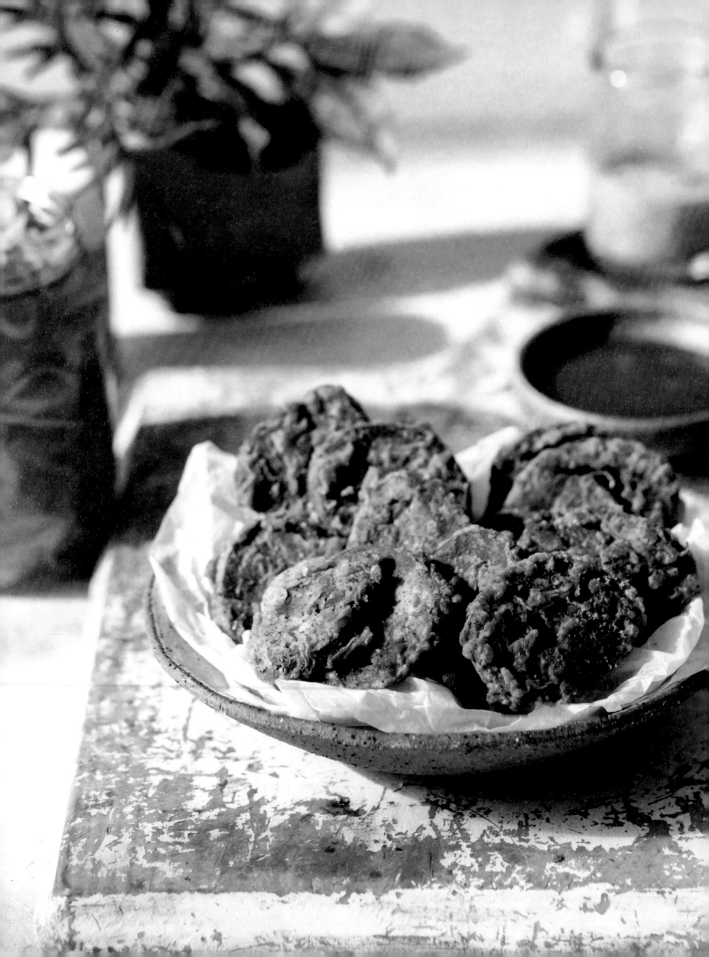

# Sous Vide Heart

I love heart. Bet you saw that one coming. No, seriously, including heart in your diet offers several impressive benefits. Heart meat is quite rich in folate, iron, zinc, and selenium and is a great source of vitamins $B_2$, $B_6$, and $B_{12}$, all of which have a cardioprotective effect, meaning they protect against heart disease. In addition, heart is rich in coenzyme Q10 (CoQ10), a fat-soluble vitamin essential for the production of ATP (adenosine triphosphate, the body's energy currency) and a big booster for cardiovascular performance. This is all based on a concept often called "the doctrine of signatures." Certain foods can be good for specific organs that look like that food or that even *are* that food. For example, walnuts, which resemble a tiny brain, are good for cognitive function; avocados, which look a bit like gonads (if you squint, I suppose) are apparently beneficial for male and female reproductive function; a sweet potato, shaped like a pancreas, can support healthy insulin function; and a heart is good for, well, your heart!

But heart can also be *exhausting* for your jaw muscles, which I suppose *could* give you a good cardiovascular workout from all that chewing. Joking aside, heart meat is notoriously tough. Yet again, here comes the sous vide technique to the rescue. It turns out a generously long sous vide can soften any heart (sorry, I couldn't resist), and, when paired with a final slicing, dredging, and frying, can render a heart melt-in-your-mouth good. And what's not to love about a melted heart?

1. Preheat the sous vide bath to 185°F.

2. Trim the beef heart of all ventricles and any silver skin on the exterior.

3. Season the trimmed beef heart by rubbing it down with sea salt, pepper, garlic powder, and, if desired, cayenne.

4. Add the heart, rosemary, thyme, and fat or oil of your choice to sous vide bag and seal it.

5. Place the heart in the sous vide bath and cook for 18 hours.

6. Remove the heart from the sous vide and thinly slice against the grain to about 1/8 to 1/4 inch thick.

7. In a bowl, lightly whisk the eggs. In a separate bowl, combine flour with seasonings to taste.

8. Dredge each slice of heart through the eggs and then through the flour. Heat a skillet over medium-high heat and pour the leftover oil from the sous vide bag into it. Place the floured heart in the skillet to sear, about 2 minutes per side, or until golden brown.

9. Serve and enjoy!

*Yield:* 4 TO 6 SERVINGS

*Total Time:* 18 HOURS

**TOOLS AND MATERIALS**

Sous vide wand and sous vide bags

Large stock pot for sous vide bath

Cast-iron or stainless steel frying pan

**INGREDIENTS**

1 large beef heart (around 2 pounds)

2 tablespoons sea salt

1 tablespoon black pepper

2 teaspoons garlic powder

1 teaspoon cayenne (optional, for "kick")

2 sprigs fresh rosemary or 1 teaspoon ground rosemary

2 sprigs fresh thyme or 1 teaspoon ground thyme

1 cup butter, lard, tallow, or duck fat, softened at room temperature, or ½ cup extra virgin olive oil

2 medium or large eggs

1 cup flour of choice (I recommend seasoning the flour to taste with extra salt, pepper, garlic, paprika, and cayenne)

***Notes:*** *These heart slices taste fantastic dipped in a bit of hot mustard or horseradish sauce.*

*If you're short on time, I've gone as short as 10 hours in the sous vide water for this recipe with good results.*

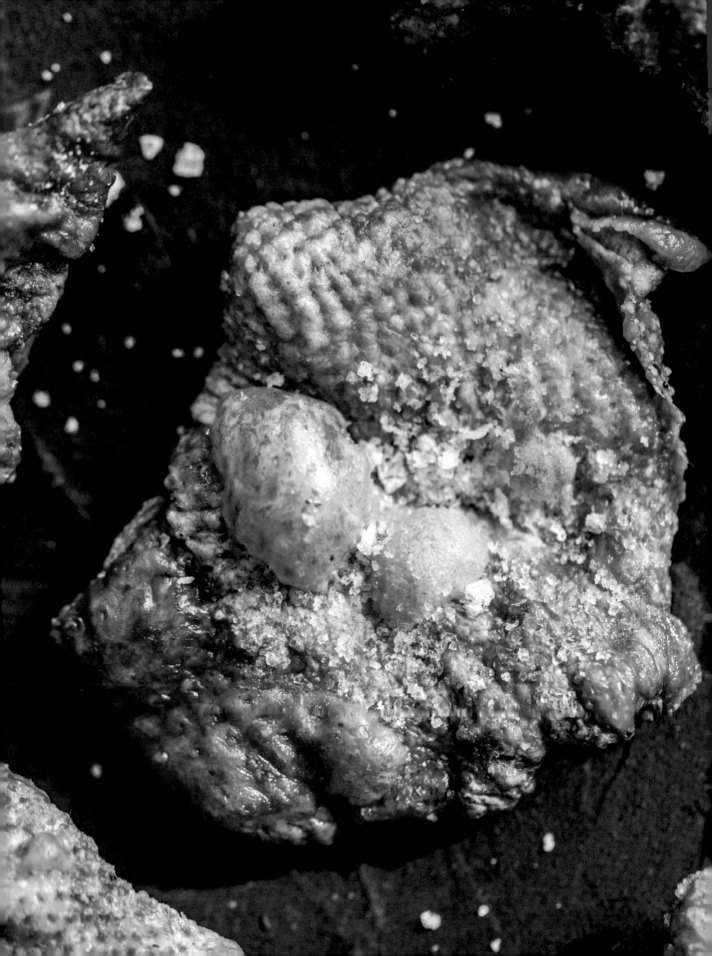

# Crunchy Chicken Cracklins

When I was a teenager, my parents used to host Iron Chef competitions, adapted from the television show of the same name, in which two chefs are pitted against each other in a meal preparation contest, often working with mystery ingredients to create an appetizer, an entrée, a dessert, or all three. When I was 16 years old, I beat my dad. I was so proud of myself. I'd finally made it. I don't even remember what I cooked. All I remember is that I beat ol' Pops.

The cooking competition tradition has now been carried forth by my own family. Every quarter or so, we host a cooking competition at our house for which I purchase the mystery ingredient, which is usually some kind of a meat-based protein, and then choose two friends or family members to be the featured chefs. Often, a chef is given a budget (usually around a hundred dollars) for grocery store supplies and extra ingredients, as well as a time deadline. We typically "unveil" the mystery ingredient around 4 P.M., and an appetizer, entrée, and dessert that all feature that mystery ingredient must be fully plated by 7 P.M. Dinner guests arrive around 6:30, and several of those guests are chosen as judges. They judge each dish based on creativity, taste, aroma, texture, and plating. Of course, we always make sure there's extra food to go around and encourage guests to bring a sharable side dish. Try an Iron Chef competition yourself sometime; it's a unique and fun way to throw a dinner party.

I happen to have been a competitor at a recent Iron Chef event that featured chicken as the mystery ingredient, and my dishes included an entrée of spicy smoked chicken wrapped in homemade tortillas with wild plant pesto, a dessert of vanilla-cinnamon Sweet Chicken Pudding (see page 140 for that recipe), and, for an appetizer, the dish you are about to discover: Crunchy Chicken Cracklins. These are prepared in the "healthy" alternative to drenching a dish in oil: the mighty air fryer. Enjoy this low-carb, keto-friendly dish as an appetizer or a side that goes well with any spicy mustard, salsa, or barbecue sauce for dipping; if you happen to be making a chicken dish anyway, this is a great way to creatively use the skin.

*Yield:* 4 SERVINGS

*Total Time:* 20 MINUTES

**TOOLS AND MATERIALS**

Air fryer

**INGREDIENTS**

An ample amount of chicken skins (skin stripped off the thighs works well)

Coarse salt

Any additional spices you'd like, such as paprika, black pepper, cayenne, or garlic, to taste

***Note:*** *You can fry these skins in a skillet on the stovetop with a heat-stable oil on medium heat, but that's messier and slightly less healthy and convenient than an air fryer. You can also bake these in the oven by laying them out on a wire rack on a baking sheet and roasting them at 400°F for about 10 minutes per side, but they just don't seem to get as "cracklin' crispy" as they do with an air fryer.*

1. Preheat the air fryer to 400°F for 5 to 10 minutes.

2. Pat the chicken skins dry with a paper towel and sprinkle them generously with the salt and your choice of additional spices on both sides.

3. Lay as many skins as possible in a single layer in the air fryer basket (don't stack 'em or they won't fry evenly) and cook for 12 to 15 minutes, flipping halfway through.

4. When the chicken skins are crispy golden brown, but not burnt, remove them from the air fryer and place them on a wire rack or paper towel to cool.

5. Repeat with additional chicken skins if you have more to prepare.

# Nature's Multivitamin Breakfast Burrito

*Yield:* 1 TO 2 SERVINGS

*Total Time:* 10 MINUTES

**TOOLS AND MATERIALS**

Large frying pan

**INGREDIENTS**

1 avocado, sliced

4 thick slices of head cheese, liverwurst, or braunschweiger

Spices, to taste (I suggest cayenne, paprika, black pepper, and salt)

1 tablespoon extra virgin olive oil, coconut oil, ghee, butter, lard, or macadamia nut oil, plus more for scrambling the eggs

2 medium or large eggs, lightly beaten

Gluten-free flour wraps (such as Siete brand), nori seaweed wraps, or 2 slices sourdough bread

A dollop of your favorite organic ketchup or salsa

1 tomato, sliced

A dollop of yogurt or sour cream

**Notes:** *I recommend ordering all three varieties of organ meat from US Wellness Meats (see Resources on page 143) and experimenting with the flavor combinations you most enjoy.*

*I personally suggest scrambled egg variations from MrBreakfast.com, Tim Ferriss's book* The 4-Hour Chef, *or, of course, the original* Boundless Cookbook *breakfast section.*

I often have a raw liver smoothie for breakfast. Yes, it sounds gross, but my recipe, Liver Lifeblood Smoothie, tastes like chocolate ice cream (see for yourself on page 105). Once you try it, you'll swear you are having dessert for breakfast and that there's no actual liver in the smoothie.

But, occasionally, I burn out on smoothies yet still desire the host of nutrients that organ meats can offer, filling me with lifeblood-like energy for the rest of the day—just like a giant, highly bioavailable natural multivitamin. So as any logical person might do, I created an idea for a nourishing breakfast burrito made out of—brace yourself—head cheese, liverwurst, and/or braunschweiger. If I've just used three terms that are outside the range of your culinary vocabulary, I'll explain.

Head cheese is not actual dairy cheese but, rather, an organ sausage that typically uses various parts of an animal's head. I order head cheese from US Wellness Meats, which includes beef tongue and heart in its head cheese, along with sea salt, onion powder, white pepper, and coriander. Just like liverwurst and braunschweiger, it is shaped like a sausage and lends itself perfectly to slicing or cubing and preparing with scrambled eggs for a mighty, nutrient-dense breakfast burrito.

Liverwurst (also known as liver sausage) is usually made from pork or beef liver and generally includes other meats and a variety of spices, depending on the recipe. It's extremely popular in many European countries. Some liverwurst varieties are spreadable, similar to a pâté, while others more closely resemble summer sausage in consistency. US Wellness Meats has a beef liverwurst that is a mixture of grass-fed beef trim, liver, heart, and kidney.

Finally, there's braunschweiger, which has a slightly milder taste than the boldly flavored liverwurst and is a mix of grass-fed trim and grass-fed beef liver. Just like the head cheese and liverwurst, it comes in a convenient sausage shape that makes it perfect for slicing and frying up in a pan with a bit of butter or olive oil for breakfast, or mixing into a breakfast burrito like the one you're about to discover.

1. Toss the avocado, sliced or cubed head cheese, and all the spices in the pan with the cooking fat or oil of your choice. Cook for 2 to 3 minutes per side over medium-high heat. I like to use a large pan for this so I can get a nice, even golden brown on the avocados and the head cheese slices.

2. Transfer the avocados and meat to a separate bowl.

3. Add more cooking fat to the pan and scramble the eggs.

4. Toss the eggs, avocado, and headcheese onto a lightly toasted flour wrap, or nori sheet, or make an open-faced breakfast sandwich by placing them on sourdough bread. Top with ketchup and a freshly sliced tomato. A dollop of yogurt or sour cream is also a perfect addition.

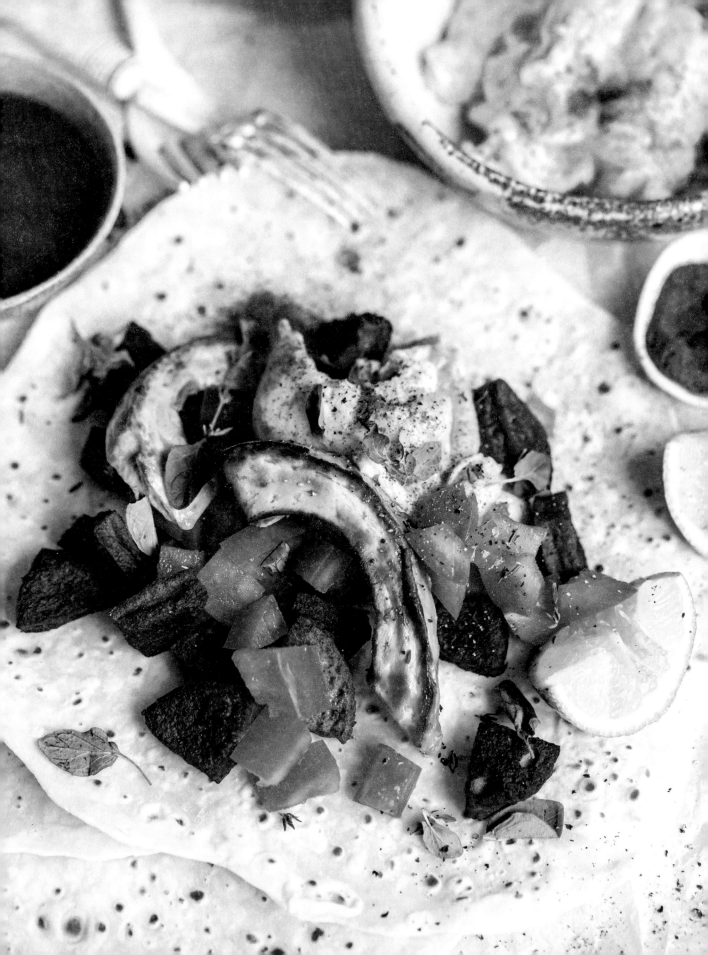

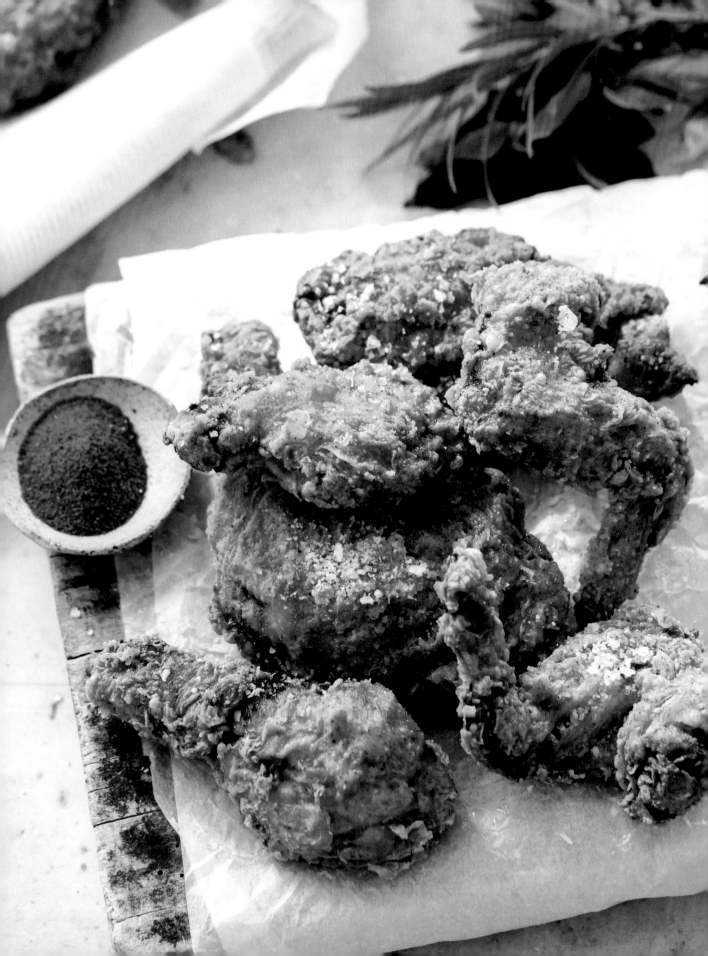

# Southern Buttermilk (Mostly) Guilt-Free Fried Chicken

*Yield:* 4 TO 6 SERVINGS

*Total Time:* 24-HOUR BRINE, FOLLOWED BY APPROXIMATELY 1 HOUR PREPARATION TIME

## TOOLS AND MATERIALS

Large Pyrex glass container or Ziploc bag

Baking sheet

Parchment paper

Large brown paper bag

Dutch oven

Oil thermometer with long probe

Meat thermometer

## BRINE INGREDIENTS

3 cups organic buttermilk

¼ cup salt

¼ cup sugar

5-pound whole chicken, cleaned and cut into wings, breasts, thighs, and legs

## FLOUR INGREDIENTS

1¼ teaspoons garlic powder

2 teaspoons onion powder

1¼ teaspoons red pepper

1¼ teaspoons chili powder

1½ teaspoons black pepper

1¼ teaspoons paprika

3 tablespoons cornstarch

2 cups Big Bold Health Himalayan tartary buckwheat flour

3 medium or large eggs

## FRYING INGREDIENTS

Enough ghee to cover all the chicken in the pot when melted

1¾ teaspoons salt

While I don't eat fried food regularly, I *do* allow myself to splurge every once in a while, especially if I'm frying the food myself and have the ability to use an oil or fat that is stable at high heat (see the table in the Resources section on page 143). And what better meal to splurge on than good ol' Southern buttermilk fried chicken, made just a bit more guilt-free by using gluten-free ingredients and no bad oils?

Furthermore, there's nothing quite so fun to do in the kitchen as putting on a good dancing song; shaking up chicken in a paper bag with cornstarch, salt, pepper, and other goodies; dredging the chicken in egg; shaking it up *again* to get a nice even coating for a crispy finish; frying it all up; and finding yourself soon mowing down on some delicious Southern-style fried chicken. Paired with homemade coleslaw and my wife's homemade freshly toasted sourdough bread (her "secret" recipe can be found in the original *Boundless Cookbook*), and you've got one delicious and traditional American meal.

The final result is a satisfying crunch on the outside and a juicy and tender texture on the inside—just how you should want your fried chicken to be.

1. Place the buttermilk, salt, and sugar in a large Pyrex glass container or Ziploc-style bag. Mix them together and add the chicken pieces. Refrigerate the chicken overnight or for up to 24 hours.

2. Remove the chicken from the brine, and discard the brine. Pat the chicken dry, season with a coating of salt, and place all the chicken pieces on a parchment- or foil-lined baking sheet.

3. Place all the flour ingredients except the eggs into a large brown paper bag and mix well. Add the chicken pieces to the flour, and shake the bag to coat the chicken.

4. Whisk together the 3 eggs in a medium bowl. Remove chicken from the paper bag and place it into the egg mixture one piece at a time. Then flip each piece to coat the other side in the egg mixture.

5. Place the egg-coated chicken back in the paper bag and shake it vigorously for about a minute to coat the chicken again. Then place each piece on a parchment-lined bake tray. Let the chicken sit to absorb the flour for 10 to 15 minutes.

6. Put the ghee in a Dutch oven over medium-high heat. Monitor with the oil temperature probe, being careful not to burn your hands. The ghee is ready when the temperature reaches 300°F.

**7.** Add the chicken pieces to the Dutch oven, and flip the chicken a few times as it cooks. Continue to use the temperature probe to maintain the oil at 300°F, which may require slight adjustments of your stove top setting. Fry the chicken for 12 to 15 minutes, or until golden brown and the internal temperature reaches 165°F.

**8.** Lay all the fried chicken pieces out on paper towels to dry, patting some of the oil away if you'd like (or place the pieces on a wire rack above paper towels) as you prepare your taste buds for a crunchy culinary experience.

*Notes:* *Should you be dairy-free and concerned about the buttermilk, please know that you won't be eating this; it's for the brine and will be discarded.*

*The next morning, this fried chicken goes great with fresh-made waffles and a drizzling of maple syrup.*

## THE HEALTH BENEFITS OF SPIRULINA

Spirulina is a nutrient-dense algae that forms tangled masses in warm alkaline lakes. Spirulina protects your cells from lipid peroxidation when you consume fried foods. Lipid peroxidation is the process by which free radicals "steal" electrons from the lipids in cell membranes, resulting in cell damage. Spirulina contains *some* amounts of the amino acid glycine, which contributes to cellular growth and health. Both spirulina and glycine also have anti-inflammatory properties and help lower cholesterol. When taken up to an hour before or after consuming vegetable oil or heated oils, these nutrients can serve to counter the cellular inflammatory effects of being exposed to lipid peroxidation. For the ultimate one-two cell-defending combo, I recommend you use a glycine powder in addition to the spirulina powder in your diet since you'll want to, optimally, consume closer to 5 grams of each when consuming potentially damaging oils.

Dr. James DiNicolantonio—author of *The Longevity Solution, The Obesity Fix*, and several other books, and a former podcast guest of mine—advises a dose of 5 to 6 grams of glycine and 5 to 6 grams of spirulina. So enjoy this fried chicken recipe, and feel free to have 5 grams each of glycine and spirulina powder afterward (e.g., stirred into a glass of pre-bedtime water) to fortify your cells—a trick that comes in handy anytime you eat fried foods.

# Crispy Fish Collars

*Yield:* 4 TO 6 SERVINGS

*Total Time:* 20 TO 30 MINUTES

**TOOLS AND MATERIALS**

Roasting or broiling pan

**INGREDIENTS**

4 to 8 fish collars, rinsed and patted dry

Approximately ¼ cup extra-virgin olive oil

Salt, to taste

1 to 2 lemons or limes, sliced, plus juice of 1 lemon

Black pepper, to taste

Fresh chopped or powdered dill, to taste

Dr. Cowan's vegetable powder of choice—enough to coat all fish in a thin layer (optional)

***Note:*** *This dish pairs well with a nice Pinot Noir and a bed of lightly salted and oiled sushi rice with a dash of chives or chopped green onions.*

Fish collar? Yep. The cut of meat from behind a fish's clavicle is hard to beat when it comes to bone-sucking succulence. Since this meat is more commonly known as *hamachi kama* (yellowtail collar) at American-Japanese restaurants, many sushi enthusiasts appreciate the existence of this buttery bite. Usually grilled or broiled, fish collars can be rendered amazingly flavorful with as little as a touch of oil, salt, and pepper, although I added just a few more goodies to this recipe.

I first discovered sea collars when they arrived at my front doorstep from Seatopia. But even though you often have to ask for them because they aren't on display at the counter, fish collars are available in many grocery stores. You can even call ahead to ask.

Once you've gotten your hands on fish collar, you can either use the simple broil recipe below or add one extra step with the *shioyaki* method. This method involves coating the fish with a layer of salt and then covering and refrigerating it for several hours or up to a day before cooking, which concentrates the flavors and texture of a fatty fish meat like collar. Fish collars often come with plenty of bones and fins. I recommend broiling them whole, then, in the same way you'd play with a lobster claw or crab leg, picking all the fatty bits of meat out from among the bones and fins so you can eat every last bit of collar goodness.

If you're consuming seafood regularly, you should also stock your pantry with sea vegetables such as nori, hijiki, wakame, arame, and kombu, all of which can pair with components such as the selenium in fish to offer a positive boost to your thyroid function. Not only are they chock-full of minerals but they may also help "sop up" some of the metals and plastics in fish and, perhaps most importantly, have a wonderful umami flavor that pairs particularly well with fish.

For this reason, I added an option to dress this recipe up with Dr. Cowan's Garden Sea-Vegetables Powder, which is a blend of dulse, wakame, and kelp, all harvested off the coast of Maine. It is certified organic and thoroughly tested for any trace of contamination by such things as heavy metals and radiation, and it offers a pleasant "oceanic" flavor that pairs well with any seafood dish. It is also fantastic added to a bone-broth soup with eggs and vegetables.

1. Preheat the broiler. Lay the fish collars skin-side down in a pan that has been drizzled with a coating of olive oil. Then coat the fish with more oil and sprinkle with salt to taste. I prefer to toss a slice of lemon or lime on top of each collar.

2. Place the pan under the broiler and broil for 3 to 4 minutes (depending on the thickness of the collars). Then flip the collars to skin-side up and broil for an additional 3 to 4 minutes, or until the skin begins to bubble and crisp.

3. Remove the fish from the broiler and season it to taste with the pepper, dill, the juice of a quarter lemon and, if desired, a generous sprinkling of Dr. Cowan's vegetable powders.

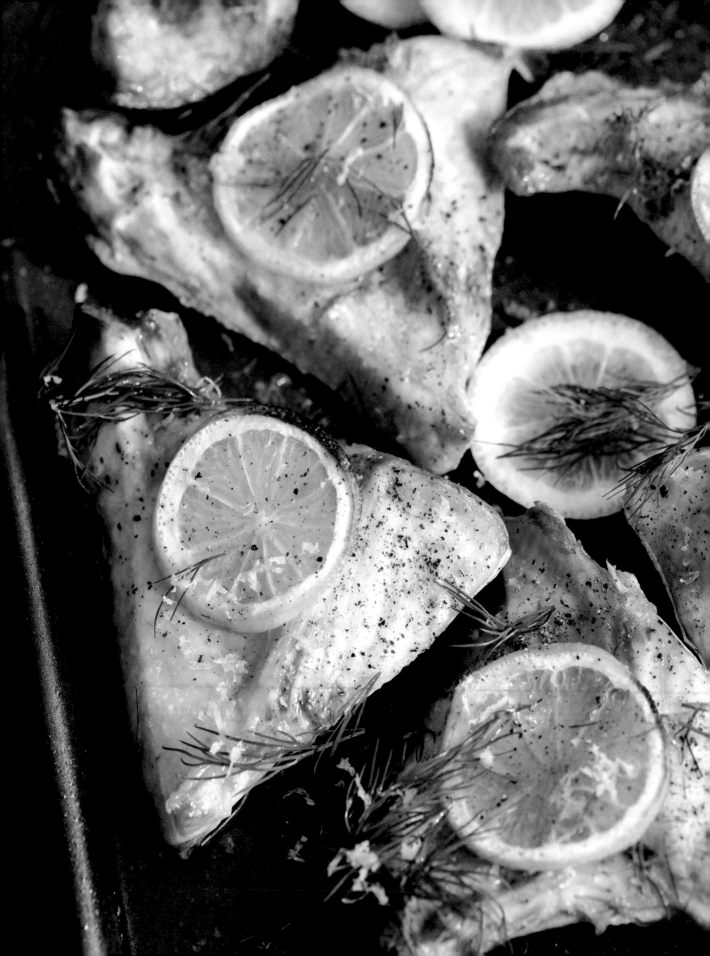

## SMASH DIET

When it comes to fish, I'm a total "SMASH diet" adherent. Choosing fish and other fat sources with a high omega-3 fatty acid composition can pay dividends for your cellular health, mitochondria, and anti-inflammatory powers.

The term "SMASH" refers to the fish that tend to be low in metals such as mercury but particularly high in omega-3s: salmon, mackerel, anchovies, sardines, and herring. SMASH fish are all small fish, and that's important because the larger the fish and the longer its lifespan, the higher its mercury content due to the accumulation of metal from eating other smaller fish.

So whenever you have the option, choose the smaller SMASH fish over larger predatory fish such as sea bass, tuna, or mahi-mahi. SeafoodWatch.org is a wonderful source for discovering which fish are sustainably sourced and low in metals.

In addition to being cleaner, SMASH fish are also rich in docosahexaenoic acid (DHA), a particularly healthy omega-3 fatty acid required for proper brain functioning. Beyond omega-3 fats, another benefit of eating SMASH fish is their favorable impact on the gut microbiome. If you're munching on the tiny, soft edible bones of these fish, such as you'd do when eating a can of whole sardines, they provide you with extra bone-building minerals.

My favorite, convenient source for my SMASH recipes is Wild Planet, which produces low-metal, sustainably sourced fish preserved in wonderful spices, marinaras, and olive oils. However, if I want a more unique but clean option that goes outside the SMASH category, such as scallops, tuna, or fish collar, I order from Seatopia, which is a healthy, sashimi-grade, flash-frozen fish delivery service.

# Reverse Sear Rib Eyes
## *with* Anchovy-Herb Compound Butter

Most steaks are cooked on a grill or in a cast-iron skillet, but a reverse sear method uses *both:* cooking the meat to perfection on a very low heat in the oven or grill and then transferring the steak to be seared in a cast-iron skillet, which creates a dark, crisp crust and unparalleled flavor.

Using a reverse sear method allows for better overall control over steak flavor and texture, and although it requires just a few extra steps, the results are far superior to simply flipping a steak a few times over some hot fire in a backyard.

When I first discovered the concept of including compound butter to pair with a reverse sear, I knew I'd upgraded my steak experience for life. It may seem fancy, and will certainly impress any of your dinner guests, but compound butter is stupid easy to make, and its many flavor combinations and herb infusions offer you a host of tasty options. One such combination is anchovies and lemons, which you wouldn't think would go well with steak, but it absolutely does. Consider this recipe to be a unique and rewarding surf 'n' turf experience.

## INSTRUCTIONS FOR THE COMPOUND BUTTER

1. Mix all of the ingredients in a bowl with your hands or a fork. Transfer the mixture to parchment paper and tightly roll it into a log shape.

2. Refrigerate for 30 to 60 minutes to solidify.

3. Cut each stick into 6 thick pats.

4. See usage instructions in steak recipe below.

## INSTRUCTIONS FOR THE STEAK

1. Cover the steaks completely with 3 pats of the compound butter (save the other 3 for later), smearing all sides of the steaks with a thick layer of the butter. Let them sit in the fridge for 2 to 3 hours prior to cooking. The steaks will absorb the flavor of the butter during this time and develop a richer and fattier flavor if you include this step.

2. Preheat the oven or grill to 275°F. Place a large cast-iron skillet in the oven or on the grill to warm.

3. Remove any butter on the steaks and dry any moisture with a paper towel. Transfer the steaks to a wire rack.

*Yield:* 2 SERVINGS

*Total Time:* 40 MINUTES, PLUS 1 HOUR TO MAKE AND CHILL COMPOUND BUTTER, PLUS 2 TO 3 HOURS RESTING TIME FOR STEAK

### TOOLS AND MATERIALS

Oven or grill

Large cast-iron skillet

Parchment paper

### INGREDIENTS FOR THE COMPOUND BUTTER

2 sticks unsalted butter, softened

6 to 8 small anchovy filets, finely chopped

4 tablespoons parsley, dried or finely chopped fresh

4 tablespoons thinly sliced green onion

2 teaspoons lemon zest

### INGREDIENTS FOR THE STEAK

2 large bone-in ribeye steaks

Compound butter, divided

Salt and black pepper, to taste

2 tablespoons avocado oil or other high–smoke point cooking oil

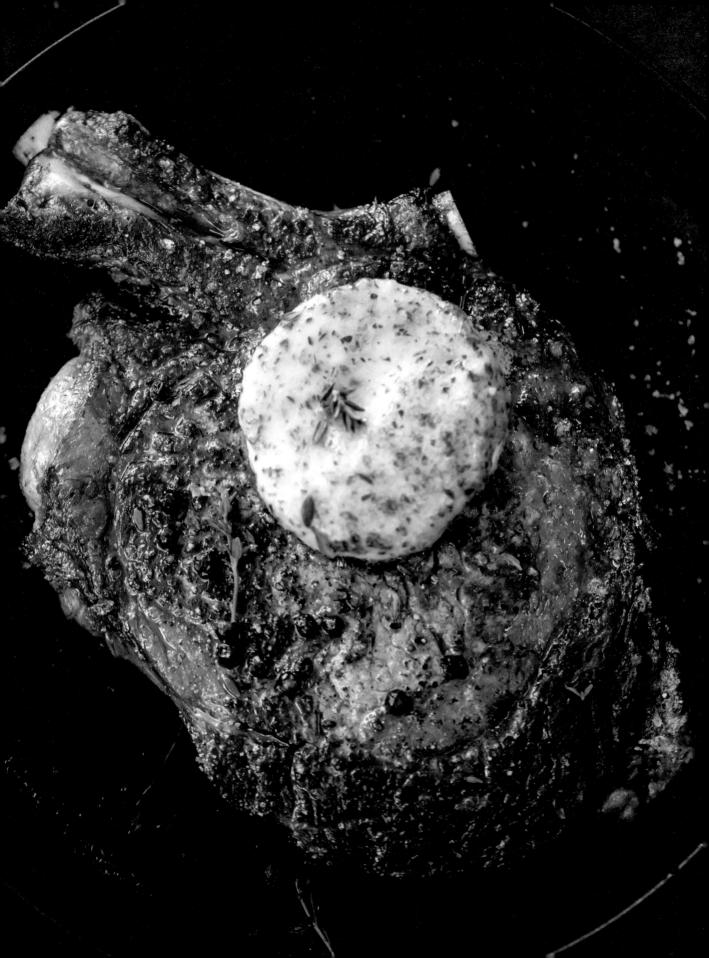

4. Generously season the steaks with salt and black pepper on both sides.

5. Place the steaks in the oven or on the grill and cook for about 15 to 20 minutes, depending on the thickness and desired level of doneness.

6. Remove the steaks from the oven or grill and set them aside.

7. Remove the cast-iron pan from the oven and transfer it to the stove top.

8. Heat the pan over high heat and add the oil.

9. Once the oil is very hot and just barely beginning to smoke, add the steaks to the pan.

10. Sear the first side until a deep-brown crust is formed, about 2 minutes.

11. Carefully flip the steaks over, top with a giant pat of compound butter, and sear an additional 1½ to 2 minutes.

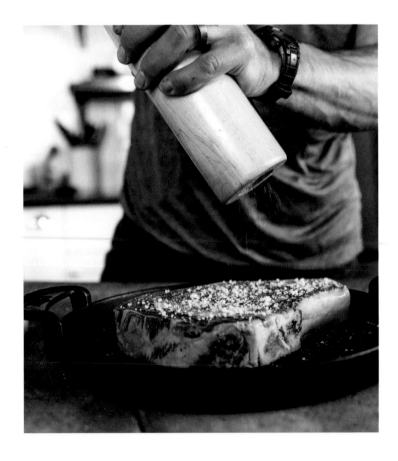

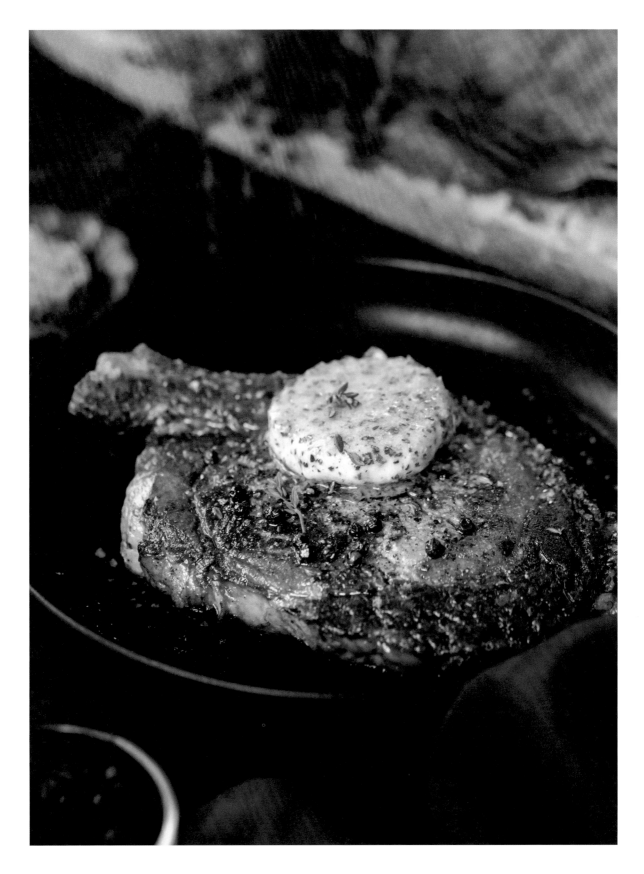

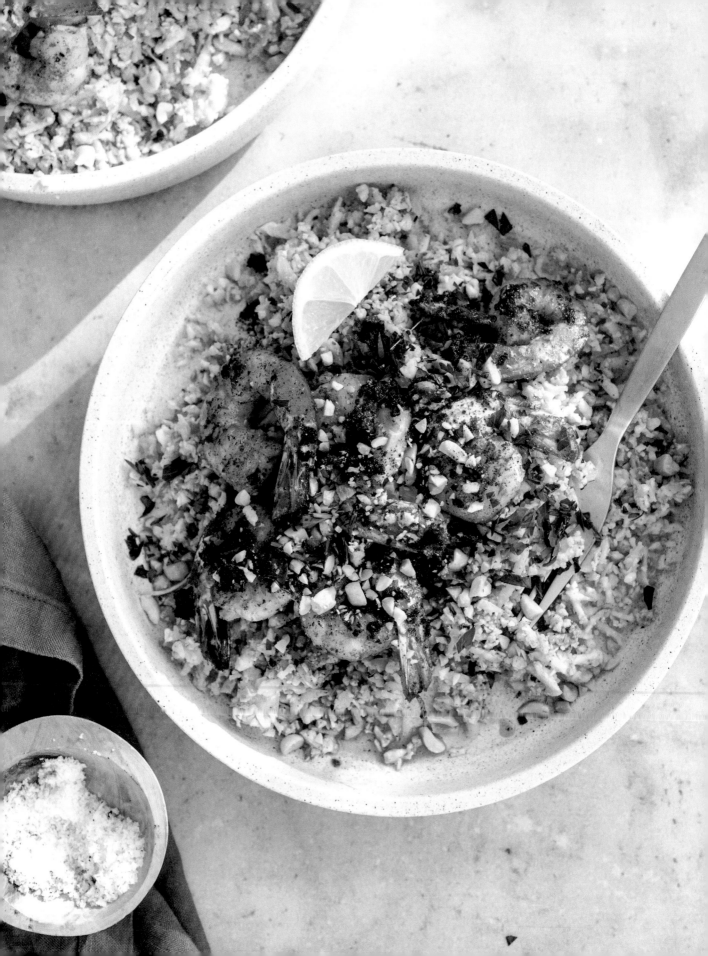

# Buttery Grain–Free Shrimp and Grits

As a bottom-feeder, shrimp can be a notoriously dirty seafood. Imported farmed shrimp can contain a host of contaminants, including antibiotics, residues from chemicals used to clean pens, and filth such as mouse and rat hair and pieces of insects. It can also be chock-full of toxic preservatives such as sodium bisulfite, sodium tripolyphosphate (STP), and 4-hexylresorcinol. So you'll definitely want to get your shrimp from a clean, sustainable source that's healthy for you and healthy for the planet too. For more on selecting and buying shrimp, see the Resources section on page 143.

Once you've got your hands on a good, clean source of shrimp, you'll be ready to try one of my fantastic grain-free, healthy comfort food recipes: shrimp and "grits," using a simple garlic-infused grass-fed butter for the shrimp and cauliflower rice as a grits substitute. The origin of this Southern comfort food is supposedly Charleston, South Carolina, where a popular breakfast dish for nearly 70 years has been fresh, local peeled shrimp fried in bacon grease with onion and green pepper, served alongside grits. While my own version would probably get me laughed at down south, it makes my taste buds smile up north, and I think you'll like it.

### INSTRUCTIONS FOR THE CAULIFLOWER RICE

1. Use a box grater, blender, or a food processor with the grater blade to blend the cauliflower into small pieces approximately the size of rice.

2. Transfer the cauliflower rice to a large paper towel or dish towel and press to remove any extra moisture.

3. Sauté the cauliflower rice in a large skillet, wok, or other pan in the olive oil over medium heat. Cover with a lid so the cauliflower can steam and become more tender. Cook for a total of 6 to 8 minutes, stirring occasionally, and then season with paprika, cayenne, salt, and black pepper. Then stir in the nut butter. Set it aside to mix with the shrimp now or refrigerate for later.

### INSTRUCTIONS FOR THE SHRIMP

1. Heat the butter in a large skillet.

2. Sauté the chopped garlic on medium-high heat in butter for 5 minutes. Toss in the shrimp along with the lemon juice, cayenne, paprika, salt, and pepper.

3. Cook the shrimp for about 2 to 3 minutes on each side, turning once midway, until the shrimp is pink and cooked through.

4. Spoon in the cauliflower rice, along with a hefty handful of Barùkas trail mix, and cook for another minute or so as you stir together all the ingredients. Alternatively, you can just serve the shrimp over the top of the rice.

*Yield:* 4 SERVINGS

*Total Time:* 35 MINUTES

**TOOLS AND MATERIALS**

Box-style cheese grater, blender, or food processor

Skillet, wok, or pan, preferably with a lid you can use to steam

**INGREDIENTS FOR THE CAULIFLOWER RICE**

I head cauliflower

2 tablespoons extra-virgin olive oil

Paprika, to taste (I use about 2 teaspoons)

Cayenne, to taste (I use about 1 teaspoon)

Salt, to taste

Black pepper, to taste

1 tablespoon nut butter

**INGREDIENTS FOR THE SHRIMP**

Butter

2 tablespoons chopped garlic cloves or 1 tablespoon garlic powder

1 pound shrimp

A few generous squeezes of lemon juice

1 teaspoon cayenne

1 teaspoon paprika

Salt and black pepper, to taste

**Note:** *I use and recommend Barùkas Butter, which features the baru nut—the nutrient-packed "super nut" also used later in this cookbook for the Barùkas Choco-Horchata (see page 92) and a star of the original Boundless Cookbook. It's jam-packed with nutrients and minerals and tastes like an addictively good mash-up between a peanut and a cashew. Barùkas also makes a trail mix that tastes great when sprinkled into this dish.*

# Ferments

It seems that the vast majority of Westerners' understanding of ferments is that this funky food group primarily consists of overpriced glass bottles of sweet 'n' sour—tasting kombucha from the local hippie health food store. But not only is the average such "ferment" more like a sugar bomb disguised as health food, it only scratches the surface of the wide world of gut-nourishing fermented compounds.

*For all resources, books, tools, and ingredients mentioned throughout this chapter, go to: BoundlessKitchen.com/resources*

On any given day, we Greenfields are eating a slice of fermented sourdough bread, topping our salad with fermented sauerkraut and carrots, wrapping fermented radishes up into a taco, and tossing a dollop of homemade fermented yogurt on top of a waffle or into a smoothie. We love to feed the critters in our guts, and you should too.

Far from being a modern, hip trend, ferments are instead a time-honored component of most ancestral human diets. The oldest fermented beverage—consisting of fermented rice, honey, and fruit—dates back to 7000 B.C. in China. Since then, the human race has experimented with fermenting grains, legumes, meat, fish, dairy, vegetables, fruits, and more. (It kind of makes me want to start a YouTube channel entitled *Can I Ferment That?*) From ancient Bulgarian yogurt to Japanese natto to Korean kimchi to Icelandic fermented shark, nearly every culture has some kind of fermented food that is included as a staple in its diet. Heck, even chocolate is technically a fermented food.

This is probably because fermentation is a handy method of preserving food that inhibits the growth of the pathogens that can spoil food. Can't eat that giant basket of cucumbers fresh from the spring garden before they rot in the refrigerator? Ferment 'em. Same for the beets, radishes, and carrots. Ever had an expensive dry-aged ribeye at a steakhouse? That idea likely originated from some ancient hunting tribe realizing they couldn't eat the whole moose in just a few days, and alas, Frigidaire freezers weren't around yet. Milk turned sour? Heck, why not just feed it some sugar, let it ferment for a day, and turn it into tasty yogurt? Interestingly, fermentation can also deactivate natural plant defense mechanisms, such as glycosides; phytates; immune-reactive proteins; and fermentable oligosaccharides, disaccharides, monosaccharides, and polyols (FODMAPs), allowing many with sensitive guts to still be able to consume problematic foods such as grains and dairy.

But the benefits of fermentation go beyond just keeping food "fresh" or rendering it digestible. Fermented foods and beverages also:

- Support the growth of beneficial gut bacteria
- Promote bowel regularity and digestion
- Exert antimicrobial effects against pathogens
- Increase the bioavailability of nutrients in food
- Decrease gut inflammation
- Support a positive mood by helping bacteria in the gut make neurotransmitters and brain-derived neurotrophic factor (BDNF, which is like Miracle-Gro for your brain)
- Boost bone density (particularly fermented dairy products)
- Control hypertension, insulin resistance, and unhealthy levels of LDL cholesterol and triglycerides
- Boost immunity and inhibit allergic responses
- Play a role in cancer prevention
- Keep skin healthy and control acne
- Assist with detoxification of environmental toxins

In this section of the cookbook, I'll share with you several of my favorite fermented staples, and, if you play close attention, you'll see other ferments spread throughout other sections too, including a shrub cocktail with a splash of vinegar (see page 89), smoothies blended with homemade yogurt (see see page 75), and even air-fried pickles (see page 19).

## One Warning When It Comes to Fermentation

While it seems there's nothing not to love about fermentation, there is one thing that should give you pause: if you have a medical or genetic condition such as histamine intolerance, fungal overgrowth, mast cell activation disorder (MCAD), mold illness, or chronic inflammatory response syndrome, some fermented foods may worsen your symptoms. In other words, let's say you got a blood or gut test and tested high for candida, yeast, or fungus: feeding that candida with a sugary kombucha or glass of fermented grape juice probably isn't the best idea. If you are interested in learning more about such issues and how to tackle them, check out my book *Boundless*.

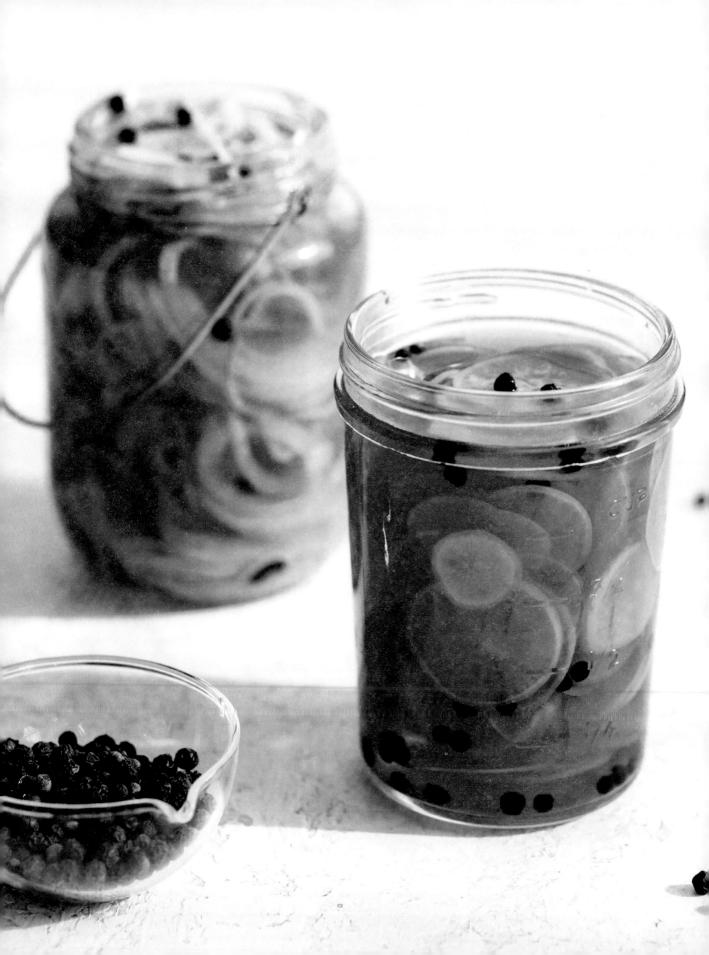

# Quick Pickled Onions or Radishes

Whenever the Greenfield family has a taco night or makes a fancy salad, we also include pickled onions, pickled radishes, or both. There's nothing quite like the sweet, satisfying crunch of a pickled onion or radish, and the bright pink and purple colors dress up just about any dish while also feeding your gut valuable bacteria and prebiotic fiber.

During canning and fermenting season late in the summer, my wife whips these up in no time flat. Sometimes she adds peppercorns or garlic cloves to the jar along with the onions or radishes to make their flavor profile more complex. It's also fine to experiment with different vinegars for this recipe, trying combinations such as a mix of white wine and rice vinegar, or apple cider vinegar and white vinegar.

1. Thinly slice the onions with the mandoline or a sharp knife and place them in a glass mason jar. Add the peppercorns and garlic clove, if using.

2. Heat the vinegar, 1 cup of water, the cane sugar, and the salt over medium heat on the stove top, stirring until the sugar and salt dissolve (about 4 to 5 minutes).

3. Remove the brine from the heat and allow it to cool for about 10 minutes. Pour it over the sliced onions. Cool the mixture to room temperature before covering your jars of onions and transferring them to the fridge.

4. Your onions will be ready to eat when they are bright pink and tender. This typically takes at least 12 hours but could take as little as 1 hour, depending on the thickness of your onions; extending the time up to 36 hours will yield even better flavor. They will keep in the fridge for up to 2 weeks.

*Yield:* APPROXIMATELY 3 CUPS

*Total Time:* A FEW MINUTES OF PREPARATION PLUS AT LEAST 12 HOURS OF FERMENTATION

## TOOLS AND MATERIALS

Mandoline (ideal but optional) or a sharp knife

Glass mason canning jars with lids

## INGREDIENTS

3 medium red onions or 20 fresh medium red radishes

10 peppercorns (optional)

1 garlic clove (optional)

1 cup white vinegar

1 teaspoon cane sugar

2 teaspoons sea salt

# Ginger–Coconut Water Kefir

A family member who will remain unnamed once said he had discovered the secret to satisfying, slippery, oh-so-easy poops. Namely, he had begun to drink several cups of water kefir per day. The topic of water kefir had come up in my podcast in the past, but I'd never gotten that into the stuff; besides, it was hard paying north of five bucks a bottle for it occasionally at a health food store (later I'd find out it cost pennies on the dollar to make gallons of the stuff, as you're about to learn). Pretty much my only kefir experience up to that point had been with *milk* kefir, which I often use as a soak or brine for cooking meats and, occasionally, in smoothies or as a milk substitute.

So I looked into water kefir. It is actually made from rice-size water kefir grains, which consist of bacteria and yeast living in a symbiotic relationship—they are not actual "grains" like oats or wheat. I purchased my first batch of water kefir grains from a company called Cultures for Health because its grains are organic, certified gluten-free, and also GMO- and dairy-free. But many folks who make their own water kefir have oodles of leftover grains and share them with friends, much like fermenting freaks who share their sourdough starters or kombucha "mothers." Water kefir is a tasty, lightly carbonated beverage that contains a host of probiotics, enzymes, and minerals that are fantastic for your gut and don't seem to feed yeast and candida like other fermented beverages such as kombucha and beer can. And, of course, there's the great poops it gives you.

Turns out, it's not difficult at all to make water kefir. All I had to do for my first ferment was add my brand spankin' new kefir grains to a large glass jar of water with a little baking soda, a touch of molasses and sugar, and a small squeeze of lime (lemon works too). I let it sit covered at about room temperature in the kitchen for five days, with occasional shaking and jar "burping" stops when I walked past the jar in the kitchen. Eventually, I strained the kefir grains out to start a new batch and refrigerated my water kefir. If cared for properly, water kefir grains can be reused indefinitely to make batch after batch like this. Later, I discovered that I could do a *secondary* ferment that allowed me to get more flavor variations. I did this by adding a fruit, spice, or herb of choice to my finished water kefir (my favorite so far has been dried ginger) and then letting that sit on the counter at room temperature for another couple of days. Finally, I learned that using coconut water instead of regular water eliminates the need for baking soda, molasses, or sugar because coconut water has all the goodies necessary for the water kefir grains to ferment beautifully.

*Yield:* 8 SERVINGS

*Total Time:* 3 WEEKS TO SOAK KEFIR GRAINS, THEN JUST A FEW MINUTES TO PREPARE, FOLLOWED BY 24 TO 48 HOURS FERMENTATION

## TOOLS AND MATERIALS

Jars (I usually use 16- to 32-ounce size)

Towel, nut milk bag, or coffee filter

Rubber bands

## INGREDIENTS

3 tablespoons water kefir grains

¼ cup sugar for soaking the kefir grains in advance

4 cups coconut water (just adjust all the values here in ingredients if you want to make more, of course!)

¼ cup dried ginger pieces or ½ cup peeled and chopped fresh ginger chunks

***Notes:*** *Should you decide to use water instead of coconut water, you can. Recipes abound online. Cultures for Health has a water kefir starter kit for less than $40 that contains everything you need to start, and it comes with good instructions too. There is also a host of helpful how-to videos and tutorials on its website, so with pretty low cost and effort, you can get water kefir into your healthy beverage rotation.*

*Water or coconut water kefir is fantastic as a liquid for making any smoothie, and it tastes pretty good as a frozen popsicle too.*

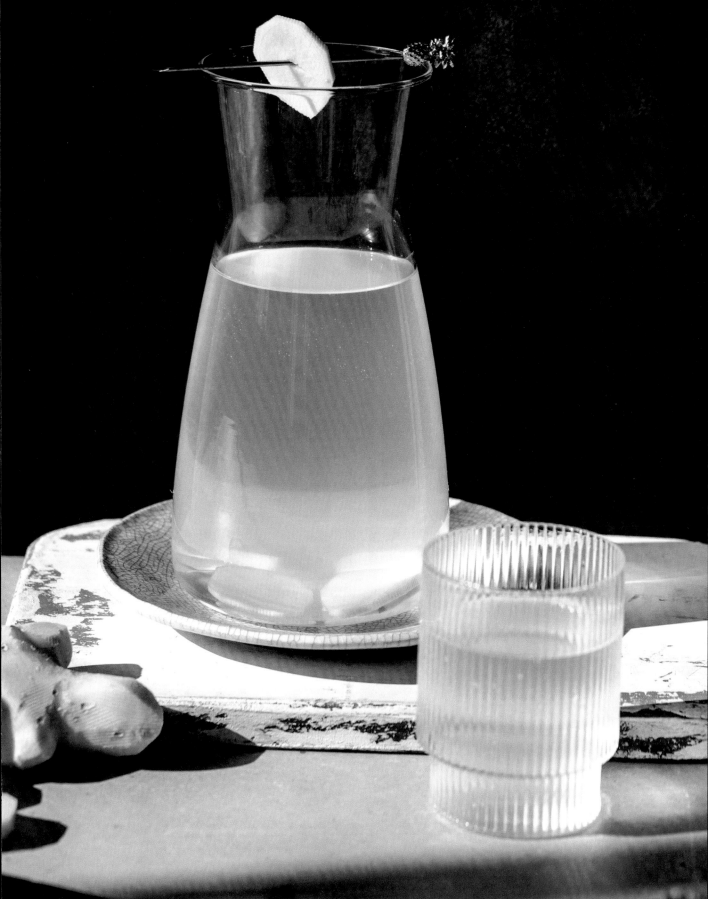

**1.** Before getting started, make sure your kefir grains are fully hydrated. You do this by soaking them in sugar water (1/4 cup sugar and 4 cups water) for at least 3 weeks. You can use that same sugar-to-water solution ratio to keep your kefir grains "fed" in between making coconut water kefir batches.

**2.** Place the water kefir grains in the coconut water. Cover the jar loosely with a towel, nut milk bag, or coffee filter secured with a rubber band.

**3.** Culture the coconut water for 48 hours at room temperature. Then strain out the kefir grains.

**4.** To add ginger flavoring (or whatever other flavoring you desire, such as blueberries, vanilla, or cinnamon), purée the ginger in a blender with the finished water kefir and then leave it out to ferment for another 24 to 48 hours, or until it's nice and fizzy.

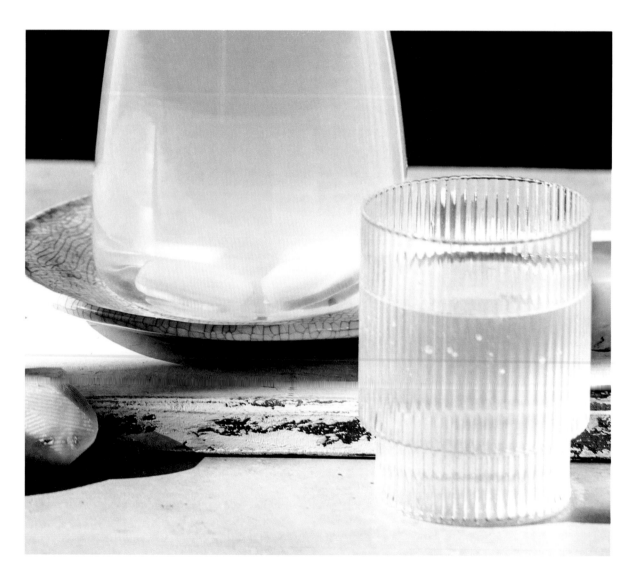

# Gut-Healing Super Yogurt

Dr. William Davis, a multi-time podcast guest of mine, first introduced me to his unique Gut-Healing Super Yogurt when I interviewed him about his fantastic book, *Super Gut*. I now use this yogurt as an ice cream or sour cream substitute, a creamy smoothie ingredient, and simply a pre-bedtime snack, often with a few chunks of dark chocolate or gluten-free granola thrown in.

So why does this yogurt work so well, especially for nourishing the tummy and even fixing problematic gut issues? The key to this yogurt's healing power is that it is fermented with several unconventional strains of a probiotic called *Lactobacillus reuteri*, which produces effects that include smoothing of skin wrinkles (due to an explosion of dermal collagen), accelerated wound healing, reduced appetite, increased testosterone and libido, bone density preservation, deeper sleep, and even—due to *L. reuteri*'s triggering of a release of the "trust and love" hormone oxytocin—increased empathy and desire for connectedness with other people. Oxytocin is also a hormone that is proving to be the key for substantial age-reversal and health effects.

Importantly, this yogurt can also be key for prevention of small intestinal bacterial overgrowth (SIBO). Telltale signs of SIBO include fat malabsorption (fat droplets in the toilet), food intolerances (histamines, legumes, fructose, FODMAPs, nightshades, and more), or health conditions such as restless leg syndrome, irritable bowel syndrome, or fibromyalgia. In most cases, to eradicate it you have choices that include using conventional antibiotics such as rifaximin that your doctor can prescribe or herbal antibiotics, two of which have some clinical evidence for SIBO efficacy (Candibactin AR/BR and FC Cidal with Dysbiocide).

But Dr. Davis discovered that a properly curated collection of microbes could be fermented to high counts by using prolonged fermentation in a yogurt recipe to obtain around 250 to 260 billion counts, or CFUs, per ½-cup serving, which is a massive amount of probiotics. For this gut-healing version of the yogurt, Dr. Davis uses three special bacterial species: *Lactobacillus gasseri*, which colonizes the small intestine and produces up to seven bacteriocins, a virtual bacteriocin powerhouse (bacteriocin contain antimicrobial peptides produced by bacteria, which can kill or inhibit bacterial strains); *L. reuteri*, which colonize the small intestine and produce up to four bacteriocins, including the powerful reuterin; and *Bacillus coagulans*, which produces a bacteriocin that also significantly assists with eradicating SIBO.

For gut healing, Dr. Davis recommends fermenting these three strains in a milk medium for about 36 hours and then consuming ½ cup per day for at least four weeks. He reports that of around 30 people who have tried this approach, 90 percent have normalized breath hydrogen gas levels and obtained relief from SIBO symptoms. Given that the best in conventional health care with antibiotics has a track record of effectiveness of around 50 percent, this is quite spectacular.

*Yield:* 8 TO 10 SERVINGS

*Total Time:* ABOUT 1 HOUR TO PREPARE, 36 HOURS TO FERMENT, AND ANOTHER 6 HOURS IN THE FRIDGE TO SET

## TOOLS AND MATERIALS

Yogurt maker (alternatively, you can use an oven or a food dehydrator)

Bowl

Thermometer

## INGREDIENTS

½ gallon goat's milk or coconut milk

2 tablespoons prebiotic fiber (inulin powder)

1 capsule *L. gasseri* BNR17

1 capsule *B. coagulans* GBI-30,6086 or 1 capsule Thorne Bacillus Coagulans

10 tablets *L. reuteri*, crushed, or ⅓ cup *L. reuteri* yogurt from a previous batch

2 tablespoons grass-fed, organic gelatin

***Note:*** *L. gasseri BNR17 is available from Mercola's Marketplace and Cutting Edge Cultures.* B. coagulans *GBI-30,6086 is available at most big box stores as Schiff Digestive Advantage. L. reuteri is available from BioGaia Gastrus.*

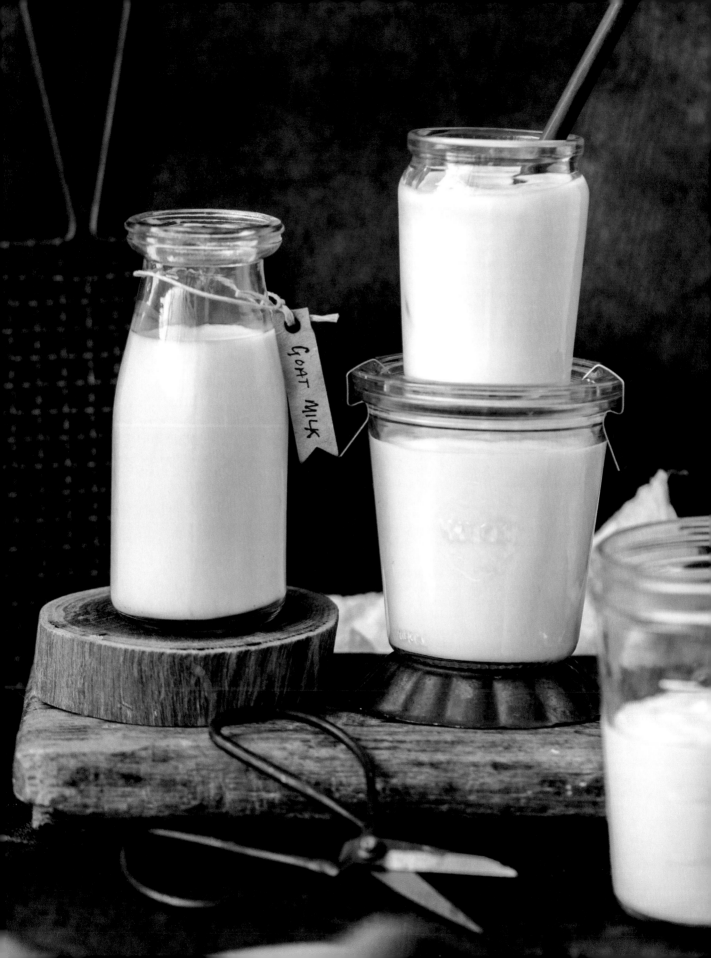

GOAT MILK

I have prepared this yogurt using goat's milk (which, for many people, tends to be a more digestible form of dairy than cow's milk) and coconut milk. It seems that most people with gut issues prefer the dairy-free option, but it's really up to you, and there are a variety of modifications to this recipe using different styles of milk and thickeners that you can find on the Internet and that I'll direct you to in the Resources section (see page 143). Below, I'm sharing my favorite way to make this yogurt. Although it's an optional step, after preparing the yogurt, while it is still warm, I recommend stirring in powdered grass-fed gelatin that you've dissolved first in a small amount of cold milk and then allowing the yogurt to cool in the refrigerator so the gelatin thickens.

1. Before you begin, it is important to sterilize any glass jars, lids, and any utensils you use in boiling hot water. You can do this by boiling a kettle of water and soaking the equipment in the hot water for a minute or two.

2. The overall process is really quite simple: you'll be combining 10 crushed Gastrus tablets, contents of one capsule of the L. gasseri and B. coagulans, prebiotic fiber, and milk, then stirring together and fermenting 98° to 100°F for 36 hours.

3. Pour the milk into a large, clean saucepan.

4. Place the saucepan on the stove top and heat the milk to 180°F. You can use a thermometer for an accurate reading.

5. Hold the milk at this temperature for 20 to 30 minutes, if possible, as the result of a longer heating time will be a better yogurt texture.

6. Remove the saucepan from the stove.

7. Cover the milk and let it cool to below 107°F. You can speed up cooling by filling a sink or bowl with cold water and setting the saucepan of heated milk in the cold water. Temperatures above 109°F will kill the L. reuteri strains, so make sure it gets lower than that. As the milk cools, a layer of skin will form on the top, which you don't need to discard.

8. Pour the milk into the yogurt-making jar(s) or other glass jar.

9. Add the prebiotic fiber and mix or whisk for 20 to 30 seconds.

10. Add the three strains of probiotics by crushing the BioGaia Gastrus tablets and opening the other two probiotic capsules, or add ⅓ cup of yogurt from your previous batch. Mix or whisk again for 20 to 30 seconds.

11. Put the lid firmly on the yogurt-making jar or jars and place them into the yogurt maker. If you're using an oven or food dehydrator instead, you can cover the jar and place it into either one.

12. Set the temperature of the yogurt maker, food dehydrator or oven to 98 to 100°F and ferment for 36 hours.

13. Remove the yogurt from the heat.

14. If using gelatin for extra thickening, mix the gelatin in a separate bowl with a very small amount (e.g., ⅛ cup) of cold or room temperature water, extra milk, or yogurt to activate the gelatin, then stir or whisk this gelatin mixture thoroughly into the warm, finished yogurt.

15. Place the yogurt in the fridge for at least 6 hours to set and then enjoy. You can also keep extra in the freezer if desired.

16. Don't forget to reserve ⅓ cup of yogurt or whey for your next batch of yogurt, which keeps you from having to use up more of the relatively spendy probiotic supplements. You can then use this mix to start your next batch rather than the probiotic capsules and tablets.

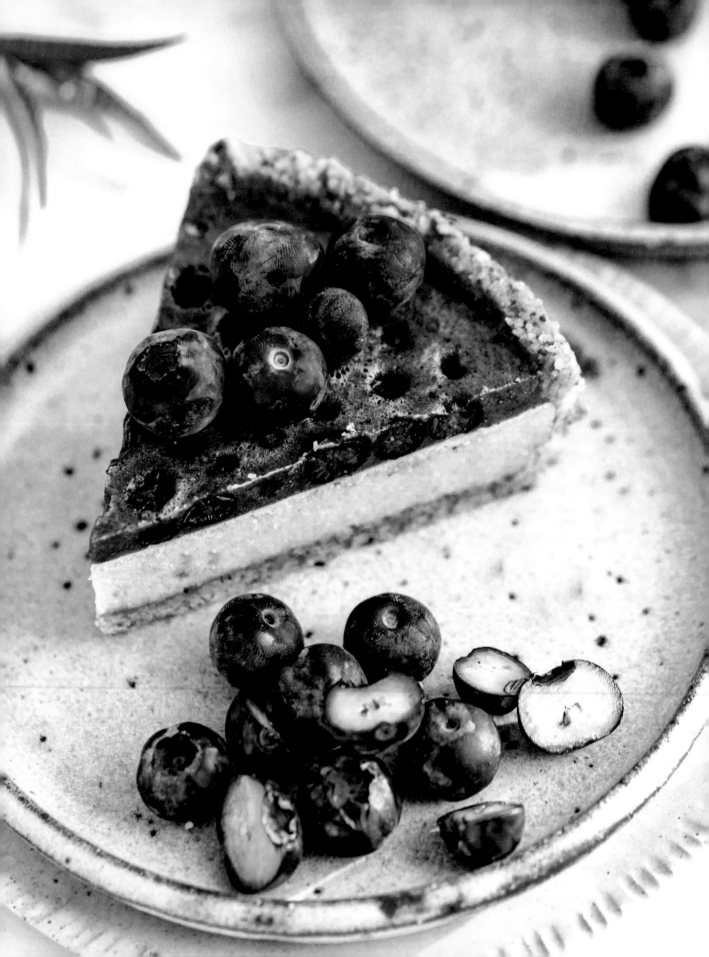

# Fermented Blueberry Cheesecake

Look: I know cheesecake is probably more fitting for the dessert section of this cookbook, but in the same way that one could *maybe* classify carrot cake as a vegetable, I'm going out on a limb and classifying this cheesecake as a healthy fermented food that I'm sticking right here in the ferments section. So there.

The first time I experienced this rich, fermented, dairy-free cheesecake, I had two revelations: 1) it's pretty much the most flavorful cheesecake I've ever had in my life (good-bye Cheesecake Factory with your 2,000-calorie sugar bombs); 2) it is an incredibly simple cake for the body to digest; and 3) due to the unique fermentation process, it doesn't leave you heavy and sedated after eating a large slice (arguably, you'll be tempted to eat many more slices than one, however).

The trick for pulling off this cheesecake properly is to use sprouted nuts, which are then given the perfect "cheesy" cheesecake flavor via the process of fermentation, which also assists with digestion due to the deactivation of many of the digestive enzyme inhibitors and antinutrients that are naturally present in nuts. The soaking and fermentation process also unlocks valuable nutrients from the nuts and makes them a rich source of probiotics.

Technically, the nuts in this cheesecake aren't really nuts. Cashews are actually a fruit and pine nuts are actually a seed (who knew?!), but both lend a perfect creaminess to this recipe that makes them the perfect pureed pair. If you want to experiment with other nuts for this cheesecake, macadamia nuts and pecans are also good choices but aren't quite as creamy. Finally, no matter which nut or seed you choose, it's important to add your sweetener *after* the nut fermentation process because otherwise alcohol and yeast can get produced, and who wants to get drunk and have a candida infection from eating cheesecake, right?

*Yield:* 1 CAKE

*Total Time:* PREPARATION TAKES 20 TO 30 MINUTES, PLUS 24 HOURS OF FERMENTATION, PLUS 6 TO 7 HOURS TOTAL CHILLING TIME

## TOOLS AND MATERIALS

Blender

Jar with cover

Yogurt maker or food dehydrator

Large mixing bowl

Springform cake pan

Colander or mesh strainer

## INGREDIENTS FOR THE FILLING

4 cups raw soaked cashews

2 cups soaked pine nuts

¾ cup melted coconut oil (make sure it's cooled down after melting but not solid)

¼ cup lemon juice

2 teaspoons vanilla extract

¼ teaspoon salt

¼ teaspoon probiotic powder/yogurt starter or 1 tablespoon of Gut-Healing Super Yogurt (see page 75)

2 tablespoons grass-fed gelatin powder

¾ cup raw honey or maple syrup, or, for a low-carb version, ¼ cup allulose or monk fruit sweetener

## INSTRUCTIONS FOR THE FILLING

1. Rinse the soaked cashews and pine nuts and place them in a blender along with 1½ cups water, ½ cup of the coconut oil, lemon juice, vanilla extract, and sea salt into a blender and purée on high speed for 60 seconds.

2. Add the probiotic powder and puree again for 20 seconds.

3. Pour the purée into a medium-size glass bowl or jar, pressing down to release any air bubbles, which keeps the surface smooth and flat.

4. Pour the remaining ¼ cup of melted coconut oil onto the surface of the purée, which seals purée and creates an anaerobic environment for better fermentation.

5. Loosely cover the jar or bowl so some air can escape and then place it in a warm, dark location or in a yogurt maker or food dehydrator set at 95 to 100°F for 24 hours, or until you see the purée become porous with air pockets.

6. Empty the purée contents into a large mixing bowl.

7. Place ¼ cup water in a small saucepan and sprinkle the surface of the water with gelatin. Heat while stirring for 60 seconds until the gelatin is dissolved.

8. Remove the gelatin water from the heat, allow it to cool briefly, and add the honey. Stir to mix.

9. Add the gelatin-sweetener mixture to the purée in the large mixing bowl and fold it in gently.

10. Once the crust is made (see below), pour the filling into the crust and smooth the surface.

11. Refrigerate for 3 to 4 hours.

## INSTRUCTIONS FOR THE CRUST

1. Place the walnuts in a blender. Pulse about 6 to 8 times until they are finely ground with as few chunks as possible.

2. Add the remaining crust ingredients and pulse again briefly a few times until an even crumble texture has formed.

3. Dump the crumble into a springform cake pan and press firmly into the bottom and about ½ inch up the sides of the cake pan.

4. Pour the cooled filling over the top of the crust and refrigerate for 3 to 4 hours (yep, that's a repeat of the instructions above; just making sure you're paying attention!).

## INGREDIENTS FOR THE CRUST

2½ cups walnuts (do not soak)

¼ cup coconut oil melted and cooled

½ teaspoon Ceylon cinnamon

1 teaspoon salt

## INGREDIENTS FOR THE BLUEBERRY TOPPING

1 tablespoon grass-fed gelatin

12 ounces frozen or fresh organic blueberries (defrost if frozen)

¼ cup honey, maple syrup, or, for a low-carb version, ¼ cup allulose or monk fruit sweetener

***Notes:*** *GI ProStart is a good brand of probiotic powder/yogurt starter.*

*I like to freeze some of this cheesecake and then cut it into small chunks and use it as a topping for a superfood smoothie. Yum!*

## INSTRUCTIONS FOR THE BLUEBERRY TOPPING

1. Place ½ cup water in a small saucepan. Sprinkle the surface with gelatin. Heat and stir for 1 to 2 minutes, until the gelatin has dissolved.

2. Fold in the blueberries and honey.

3. Take half this mix and purée it in a blender for about 30 seconds. Then pour it through a colander or mesh strainer to remove the seeds.

4. Fold this purée into the other half of the blueberry mixture so you have a mix of the thick chunky parts and purée.

## FINAL INSTRUCTIONS

1. After the cheesecake has chilled for 3 to 4 hours in the fridge, pour the blueberry topping evenly over the surface.

2. Chill for at least 3 additional hours in the fridge or overnight before serving.

## SOAKING AND SPROUTING SEEDS

Here's a quick primer on soaking and sprouting: cover your raw seeds or nuts with room-temperature water and around a teaspoon of salt for every cup of nuts. Stir well to dissolve the salt and then leave for two to four hours at room temperature to soak for a softer nut (er, fruit!), like a cashew, and overnight for a harder nut (er, seed!), like pine nuts. Next, drain with a colander or mesh strainer, rinse a few times with cool or room-temperature water, and voilà! You've got a nice, soft final product ready for puréeing and fermentation.

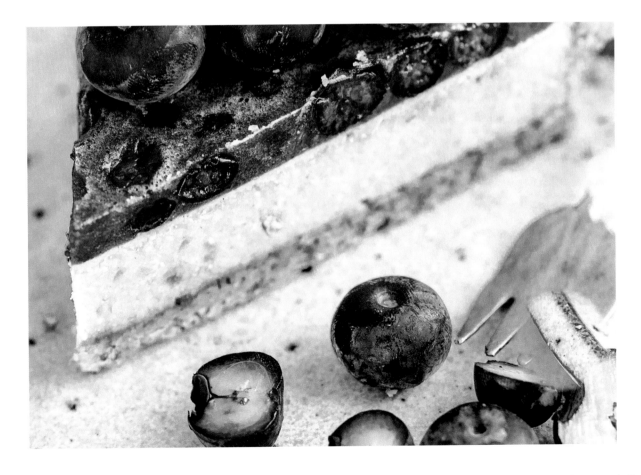

# Beverages

I drink far less water than you'd think. Sure, I've got my entire house outfitted with all the fanciest, highfalutin, double-carbon-block, vortexed, structured water filtration technologies—but plain ol' water? I just don't drink much of the stuff. Sure, I begin each day with a giant 32-ounce mason glass jar full of pure, clean, filtered water, but I add electrolytes, hydrogen, vitamin C, and even sometimes a squeeze of lemon or splash of apple cider vinegar to the water (see Ben's Biohacked Morning Cocktail, page 85).

*For all resources, books, tools, and ingredients mentioned throughout this chapter, go to: BoundlessKitchen.com/resources*

Throughout the day, in addition to chewing natural gum such as Turkish mastic gum, I drink organic coffees and teas, stevia- or monk fruit–sweetened soda, oodles of sparkling water, canned kava beverages, natural energy drinks, coconut water kefir, water with extra minerals squeezed into it, and low-sugar kombucha. At dinner I drink organic dynamic wine, or a fresh cocktail made with bitters, or ketones, or fresh juice mixed with sparkling water.

Fact is, even without sticking to plain water, you can keep your appetite satiated between meals, stay hydrated, and make hydration tasty and fun, especially if your beverages of choice don't include categories such as sweet soft drinks, sodas laden with artificial sweeteners, or mixed alcohol drinks full of high-fructose corn syrup and the like.

As an example, let's look at the diet of those living in Blue Zone longevity hot spots. With very few exceptions, people in Blue Zones consume four types of beverages throughout the day: water, coffee, tea, and wine. Usually, they drink coffee for breakfast, tea in the afternoon, wine in the evening, and water all day. In these populations, there appear to be health and longevity benefits derived from all the extra vitamins, minerals, and nutrients one gets from consuming a variety of beverages in addition to plain water. So my theory is: why not upgrade your water too?

So say good-bye to plain ol' water, and say hello to some of my favorite daily and nightly beverages, brews, and cocktails.

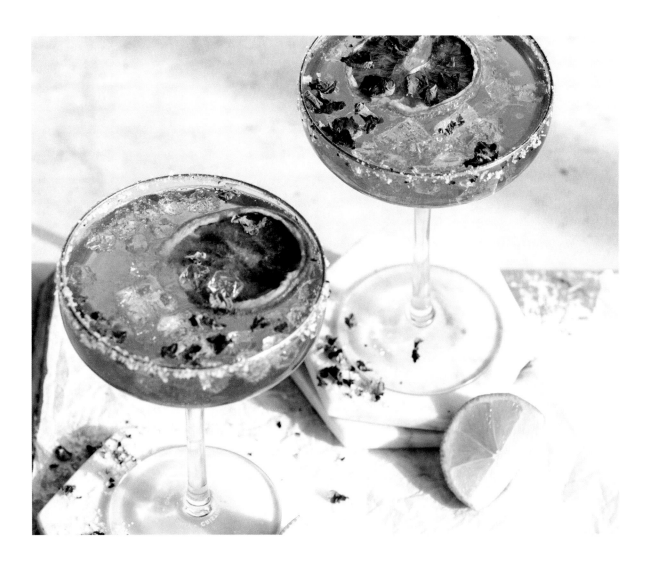

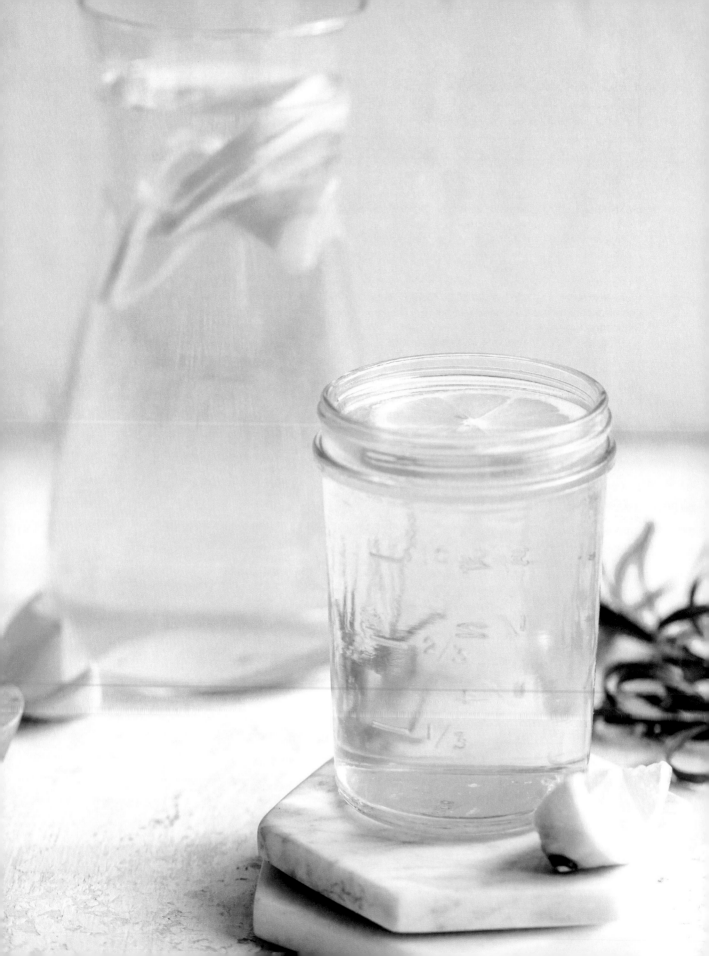

# Ben's Biohacked Morning Cocktail

*Yield:* 1 SERVING

*Total Time:* 2 MINUTES, PLUS A
FEW MINUTES' DISSOLVING TIME

**TOOLS AND MATERIALS**

Large glass mason jar

**INGREDIENTS**

1 to 3 hydrogen tablets

Quinton, Protekt, LMNT, or Manna

1 scoop Jigsaw Health Adrenal
Cocktail

1 teaspoon baking soda

A splash of apple cider vinegar or a
squeeze of lemon

Every morning, within 30 minutes of waking, I drink a giant 32-ounce mason glass jar jam-packed with hydration, minerals, adrenal support, antioxidants, and immune boosters. The ingredients I use for this "cocktail" are easy to travel with, and anyone I've turned on to this brew reports significant improvements in energy and mental function throughout the morning.

The first ingredient in this water is minerals or electrolytes. For this, my favorite option is Quinton, which is a highly concentrated and purified marine plankton bloom extract (sounds sexy, right?) that is extremely close to human plasma in terms of its actual chemical composition. It basically tastes like drinkable seawater. Since the hypertonic version of Quinton is best for energy and wakefulness, I use one serving of that concentration for my morning drink. But if I repeat this drink in the late afternoon, which I often do, I use the isotonic version of Quinton, which is a bit more relaxing. Alternatively, if you want to experiment with different flavor combinations of electrolytes, or use options that are less expensive than Quinton, a few other good brands of electrolytes include Protekt (liquid), LMNT (powder), and Manna, which is also good for coffee; it's a dark black liquid with a few added goodies, such as shilajit, fulvic acid, and microminerals.

The second ingredient is molecular hydrogen tablets. Hydrogen is a selective antioxidant with thousands of peer-reviewed studies showing it attenuates oxidative stress, improves cellular function, and reduces chronic inflammation. I typically dissolve three hydrogen tablets into my drink for 3 to 4 minutes and then drink the dissolution soon after (within 5 minutes) so that the hydrogen gas doesn't dissolve off the top of my water.

The third ingredient is a heaping scoop of Jigsaw Health Adrenal Cocktail, which provides even more minerals, along with a hefty dose of vitamin C for adrenal support and immune function. When I use this, I also add a small amount of baking soda (slightly less than a teaspoon) to balance out the acidity of the ascorbic acid and to increase the absorption of the vitamin C. If I don't happen to have the Adrenal Health Cocktail on me, I'll instead often use a splash of apple cider vinegar or a squeeze of about half a lemon. Adding all this to the brew also seems to help quite a bit with bowel regularity later in the morning, so there's an added bonus for you.

**1.** Thinly slice the onions with the mandoline or a sharp knife Stir all ingredients into the large glass mason jar with room-temperature or slightly warm water. Wait a few minutes for the hydrogen tablets to fully dissolve and then chug it all down (or sip slowly) and enjoy!

# Shroomie Tea

About an hour after I've had my Biohacked Morning Cocktail (see page 85), I spend the first 45 minutes or so of my work day sipping on some kind of fancy, warm brew, which can vary from organic coffee with a pinch of salt and drops of stevia to foamy, blended medicinal mushroom extracts to spicy cayenne cacao tea. I drink this particular brew so often that I simply had to include the recipe here.

Now, you may associate "shroomies" with the magical mushroom variety of fungi, aka psilocybin, but that's really not what this tea is all about. Instead of the magic variety of mushrooms, this recipe calls for the type of medicinal mushroom supplements you can find in nearly every health store. For thousands of years, mushrooms have reigned supreme as a powerful source of nutrients for physical and mental strength, and they can now be grown, harvested, and processed with low ecological impact. But it's important you choose a mushroom that was grown in a way that mimics the natural growth cycle of the mushroom from beginning to end.

See, all fungi grow from decay, absorbing nutrients through a rootlike structure called mycelium and sprouting a fruiting body above the ground. The fruiting bodies then release the fungi's reproductive spores, and a whole new life cycle begins. Fruiting bodies come in all different shapes and sizes, which is why we have the fuzzy-ish morel, the shiny, glossy reishi, the brain-like lion's mane, and the kaleidoscopic turkey tail.

Inside the cell walls of fungi are large molecules made of multiple sugar molecules. These are called beta-glucans and are just one of the components that make mushrooms so healthy, acting like soluble fiber (if they are properly extracted) to nourish the digestive tract. Fungi also contain vitamins B and D, folate, antioxidants, and, quite notably, a host of immune-boosting compounds.

If you're lucky enough to harvest mushrooms yourself, you'll likely be getting pure mycelium extracts, a term used to define a fungus that absorbs nutrients from its natural environment. A mushroom grown in its natural habitat, such as on the forest floor or on a log, is quite rich in enzymes and beta-glucans but harder to get your hands on if you live in an urban setting.

Next, there are mycelium on grain (MOG) mushroom products, which are derived from fungus grown on a grain such as rice, oats, and corn. Many claim that growing mushrooms on grain is an appropriate substitute for a mushroom's native growing conditions, but the problem is that grain is filled with starchy polysaccharides that deprive the fungi of the normal decay they would get from their natural substrate and cause the fungi to absorb starches from the growing grain substrate. This extra starch can create false-positive tests for healthy, bioactive compounds in mushrooms, so companies often add back synthetic beta-glucans to make the product seem healthy when it's nowhere near as good as mushrooms grown in a native environment. I recommend you avoid any commercial mushroom product that lists anything

*Yield:* 1 SERVING

*Total Time:* 5 MINUTES

**TOOLS AND MATERIALS**

Latte frother

**INGREDIENTS**

1 to 2 teaspoons your choice of powdered mushrooms

A pinch of salt

A sprinkling of Ceylon cinnamon

Stevia, to taste

1 piece organic dark chocolate, crumbled (optional)

Hot water or your milk of choice

**Note:** *For stevia, I recommend Omica Organics vanilla or butterscotch. For powdered mushrooms, I recommend Four Sigmatic mushrooms, particularly cordyceps, chaga, lion's mane, the 10-Mushroom Blend, or a blend of any.*

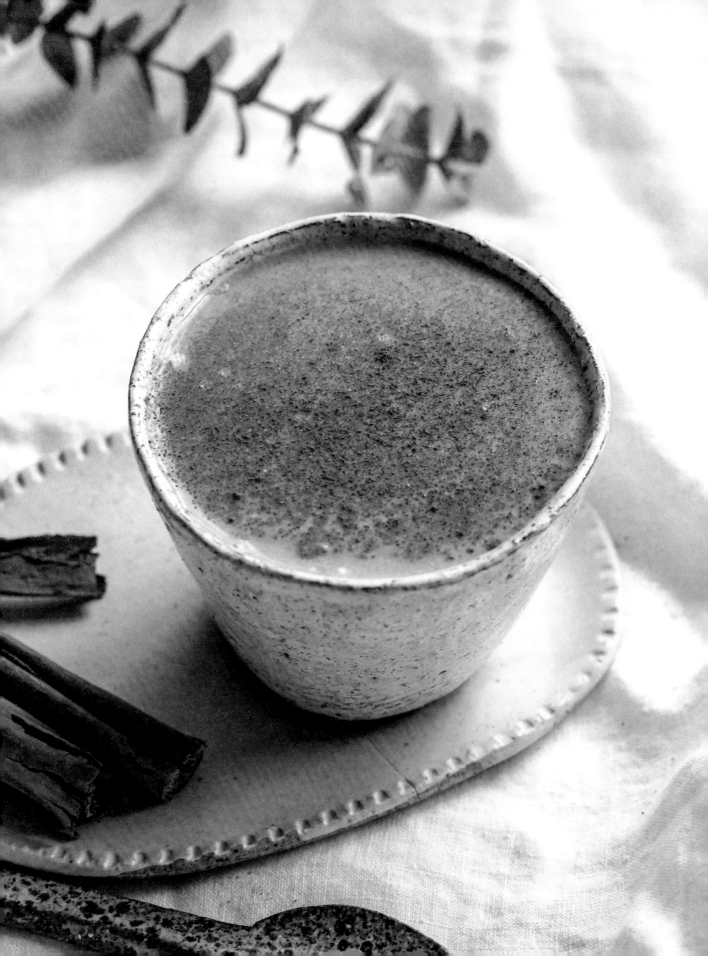

like the following as an ingredient: myceliated grain, mycelial biomass, cultured oats, freeze-dried myceliated brown rice.

Finally, there are whole fruiting body extracts, made through a process in which the whole fruiting body from mushrooms is extracted from fungi grown on a natural hardwood substrate that closely mimics nature. Chaga, for example, can be grown on a native birch log, harvested at the point of its life cycle during which the medicinal properties are the most potent, and gently processed using steam or hot water to crack open the cell walls and release the beta-glucans tucked inside the cell walls. This is the best type of mushroom product to get if you're not harvesting your own.

Once you have mushrooms of the whole fruiting body variety, the recipe is really quite simple. This also serves as a low-calorie "pre-workout" beverage, since I'm typically sipping this brew around 6 A.M., then hitting the gym around 8:30 A.M., and having breakfast around 10 A.M.

1. Put the powdered mushrooms, salt, cinnamon, and stevia into a large mug.

2. If you're seeking a more calorie-dense beverage treat, stir in dark chocolate prior to the frothing process.

3. Pour in the hot water, and as you pour, use a latte frother to get your brew nice and bubbly.

4. Sip slowly and savor!

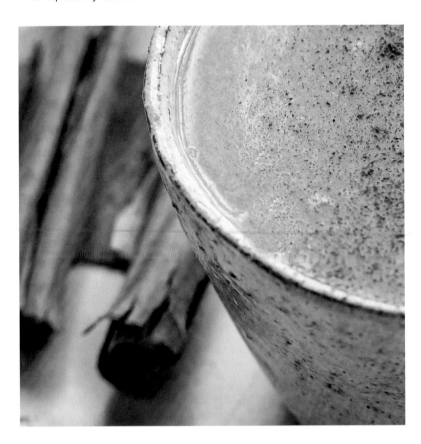

# Shiso Shrub Fusion

If you saw my vinegar deglazing instructions in the meat section of this cookbook (see page 41), you're already familiar with T. J. Robinson, my friend who travels around the world hunting down the best of the best extra-virgin olive oils and artisanal vinegars. When I interviewed him on my podcast, we had a fascinating discussion about the unique fermentation process of vinegar preparation, how to taste and select the finest of vinegars, and, quite notably, vinegar's host of health effects.

For example, vinegar can lower blood sugar, particularly when paired with a meal rich in carbohydrates, making it the perfect companion to a dinner party or addition to a cocktail. One theory is that vinegar interferes with the digestion of carbohydrates by blocking enzymes that break down carbs, resulting in less of a blood sugar spike after eating and a greater feeling of fullness. This is why I often recommend folks throw back a shot of apple cider vinegar before diving into a feast or other carbohydrate-rich meal.

Furthermore, the acetic acid in vinegar may help prevent development of abdominal fat and prevent excess fat storage in the liver. Vinegar also contains a host of polyphenols, plant chemicals that have an antioxidant effect that may protect cells from oxidative stress, which is a possible stimulator of tumor growth. This is a possible reason why vinegar seems to prevent the growth of cancer cells or cause tumor cells to die in cell and rodent models. Certain vinegars like apple cider vinegar also contain pectin, which can act as a prebiotic fuel for beneficial bacteria. Vinegar can also be used to treat gastroesophageal reflux disease (GERD) because it may increase stomach acid and improve digestion, while possibly also lowering blood pH to a more acidic environment that destroys harmful pathogens in the gut.

But perhaps most importantly, vinegar is a low-calorie, nutrient-dense way to enhance the flavor of just about any food or drink, including a shrub cocktail. A shrub is a nonalcoholic syrup typically made from a combination of concentrated fruits, aromatics or bitters, sugar, and vinegar. When mixed with ingredients like soda or tonic water and your favorite alcohol (an optional step, and, yes, I often use my shrub with soda water as a mocktail), the result is a "healthy" cocktail that's fun to drink and easy to make. For this particular shrub recipe, I like to use shiso leaves, which are an aromatic herb from the same botanical family as mint. You may have tasted shiso before at Japanese restaurants because it's a digestion-enhancing, flavorful garnish that traditionally accompanies sushi and sashimi. Year-round I grow and harvest my own shiso leaves indoors using a vertical gardening setup in my garage called a Lettuce Grow, which is quite a handy tool to have on hand if you want access to fresh produce and herbs in any season. I include details on that at BoundlessKitchen.com/resources.

Technically, you can make a shrub syrup for cocktails and mocktails in two ways: the hot method (fresh fruit, leaves, or herbs simmered in simple syrup) and the cold method (fresh fruit tossed with sugar and left to sit for a few days). The recipe here

*Yield:* 6 TO 8 SERVINGS

*Total Time:* 1 HOUR 15 MINUTES

**TOOLS AND MATERIALS**

Large pot

Fine mesh strainer

Glass jar or bottle

Cocktail shaker

**INGREDIENTS FOR THE SHRUB (FEEL FREE TO ADJUST RATIOS IF YOU'D LIKE TO MAKE LESS)**

2 cups shredded and chopped shiso leaves

2 cups sweetener

2 cups vinegar of choice

**INGREDIENTS FOR THE COCKTAIL OR MOCKTAIL**

1 to 2 ounces spirit of your choice, such as vodka, gin, whiskey, tequila, or rum (omit for a mocktail)

Ice (optional)

Mixer of your choice, such as club soda, tonic water, or juice

Garnishes of your choice, such as lime wedges, blueberries, or other fruit

***Notes:*** *For sweetening, most shrub recipes use ample amounts of agave syrup, but I prefer a lower-sugar, lower-carb option such as monk fruit sweetener. But if you don't care about the carbs, you can also use white sugar, coconut sugar, or honey, or a mix of any.*

*For vinegar, I highly recommend the pear balsamic vinegar or calamansi gourmet vinegar from GreenfieldPantry.com, which you can combine with a cheaper vinegar such as white vinegar if you don't want to use too much of your spendy vinegar. The shrub can be refrigerated for up to 6 months.*

*A shrub syrup is also wonderful drizzled over a bowl of strawberry, chocolate, or vanilla ice cream.*

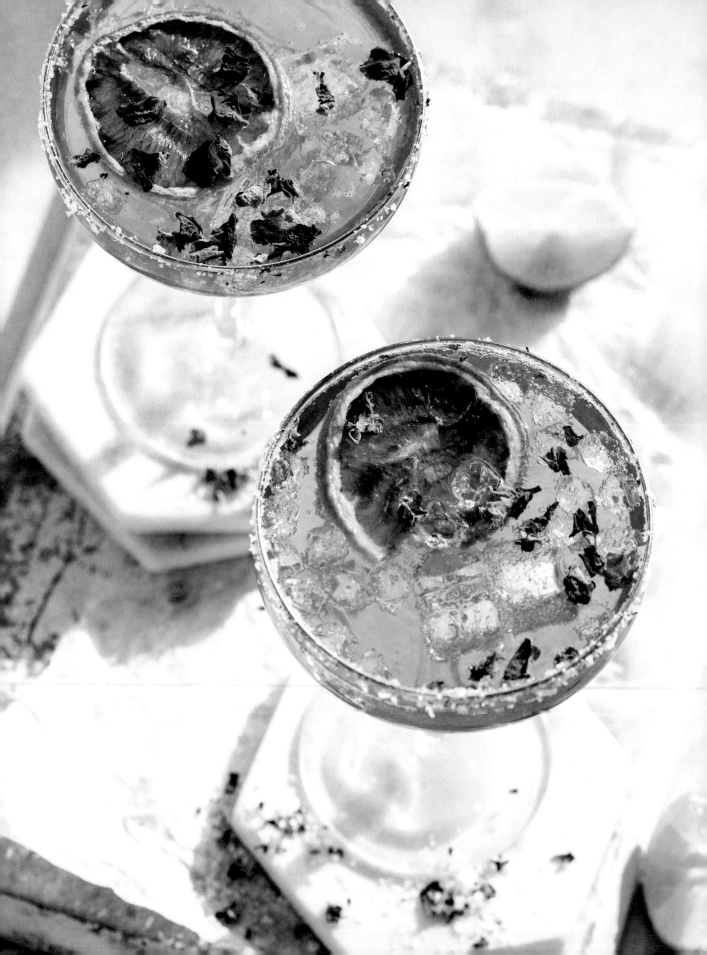

uses the hot method, which is faster, but should you decide to experiment with other ways of making your shrub syrup, you can certainly consider a cold method: let your leaves or berries of choice steep in vinegar and sweetener for two days at room temperature in a large glass jar. Then strain out the liquid and bottle it up.

Finally, proper ratios are also important for a well-done shrub. Most recipes call for an approximate 1:1:1:1 ratio of fruit, leaves or herbs, sugar, and vinegar (for example, 2 pounds chopped plants, 2 cups sugar, 2 cups water, and 2 cups vinegar), which makes it simple to make more or less shrub, depending on how much you want to have on hand to freeze or store in the refrigerator.

**1.** Place the shiso leaves, sweetener, water, and vinegar in a large pot and bring it to a boil over medium-high heat. Lower the heat to simmer and cook, uncovered, until the shrub is a deep amber and the leaves are wilted and have turned dark, which should take about 1 hour.

**2.** Strain the shrub using a fine mesh strainer, pressing on the leaves with a large spoon to extract all the liquid. Use the shrub immediately or transfer it to a glass jar or bottle, close tightly, and refrigerate.

**3.** When you're ready to make your cocktail or mocktail, combine 1 to 2 ounces of vodka, gin, whiskey, tequila, or rum and 1 to 2 ounces of shrub syrup (to taste) in a cocktail shaker with ice. Shake vigorously for about 10 seconds and then serve in a tumbler, in a martini glass, or (my preference) over a large glass of ice. Top with soda water, tonic water, or a juice of your choice (such as pomegranate or pineapple) to taste. Garnish with lime wedges, blueberries, or any other fruit of your choice.

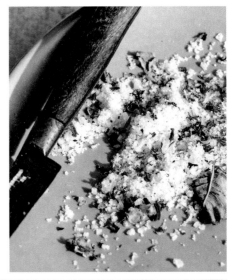

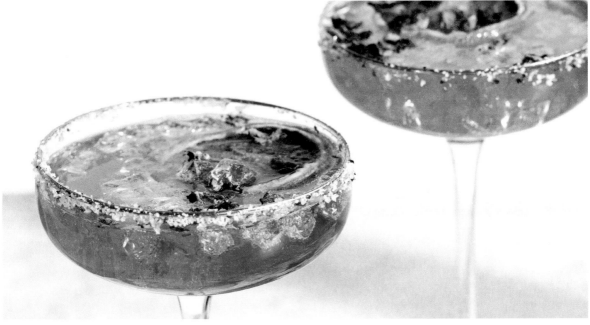

# Barùkas Choco-Horchata

As proprietors of their own cooking channel and podcast (GoGreenfields.com), my twin sons are constantly coming up with new twists on traditional recipes and go-to comfort foods, from colorful boba tea to s'more soufflés to magical cereal bars to healthy homemade dog food; their creativity knows no limits. So I wasn't surprised when they came up with a twist on one of their favorite drinks to order when we go out for Mexican food: horchata.

Horchata is a traditional Mexican drink usually made of white rice soaked in water and then flavored with cinnamon, sweetened with oodles of granulated sugar, and minced up in a blender and strained to remove the solids. Some versions of horchata are dairy-free while others use milk, and some versions include a variety of nuts or added flavors such as vanilla or coconut.

We've tried several horchata recipes with different ratios and varieties of rice, nuts, and herbs and spices, but the king of them all turned out to be a horchata made of Barùkas nuts. Ever since they were introduced to me by superfood hunter Darin Olien, Barùkas have been a staple in our household. They are pretty much the healthiest nuts on the planet—literally a mini-cocktail of hard-to-find micronutrients and plant-based protein, far easier to digest than most nuts, and perfect fuel for what my sons and I call our Barùkas Choco-Horchata.

Pair this tasty brew, warm or cold, in mugs (perhaps on a taco night using the Tongue Tacos recipe on page 33); drink as an alternative to a cocktail, such as with rum and lemon juice; pour over ice and sip as a refreshing midday beverage; or even freeze and use as popsicles or ice cream substitute.

1. Drain the soaked Barùkas nuts and place them in a blender.

2. Add the hot water and blend on high speed until the mixture is homogenous and almost smooth, about 2 minutes.

3. Carefully pour the blended nuts through a cheesecloth-lined fine mesh sieve into a large bowl or pitcher. Gather the ends of cheesecloth together and squeeze out all remaining liquid.

4. Add the sugar and salt to the horchata liquid and stir or whisk together. Cool completely and then transfer to a bottle or container and store in the refrigerator. Serve the horchata over ice, sprinkled with cinnamon, or if you prefer, warm like hot chocolate. This recipe can be stored in the refrigerator for up to a week.

*Yield:* 8 SERVINGS

*Total Time:* 24 HOURS TO SOAK, 10 MINUTES TO PREPARE

**TOOLS AND MATERIALS**

Blender

Cheesecloth

Fine mesh sieve

Large bowl or pitcher

**INGREDIENTS**

1 cup Barùkas nuts, soaked in water for 24 hours at room temperature

4 cups hot (but not boiling) water

½ cup organic cacao powder

¼ cup sugar, honey, or alternative sweetener

¼ teaspoon salt

2 teaspoons cinnamon

**Notes:** *Monk fruit is a good option for an alternative sweetener since you can use the same ratios as sugar in recipes. Also known as luohan guo, it is an herbaceous perennial vine and contains the compound mogroside, which creates a sweetness sensation 250 times stronger than sucrose.*

*Don't toss those soaked nuts once you've strained out the nut milk. This "nut pulp" can be used in a variety of ways. You can process or blend it with ingredients such as coconut, vanilla, dates, and coconut oil until you have a finely chopped consistency that's perfect for a crust; blend it with avocado, cacao powder, and sweetener to make chocolate pudding; blend it with garlic, lemon juice, olive oil, salt, and tahini to make raw hummus; use it as an ingredient in cookie batter; toss it in a smoothie with chia seeds and flax seeds for bowel-moving fiber; or even mix it up with other leftover ingredients such as spent coffee grounds to serve as a face and body scrub.*

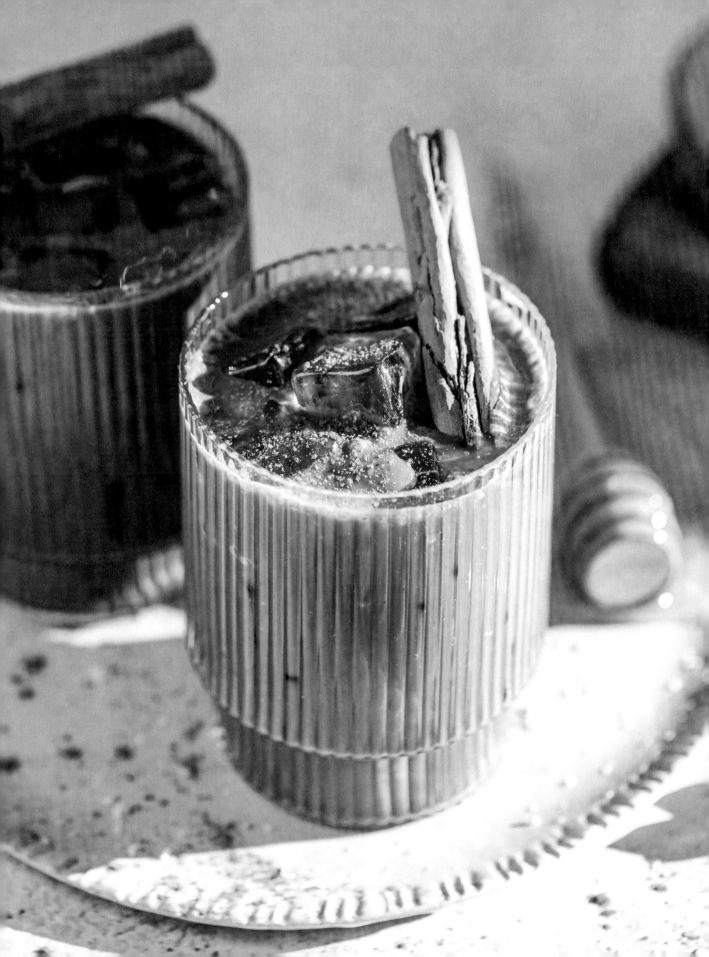

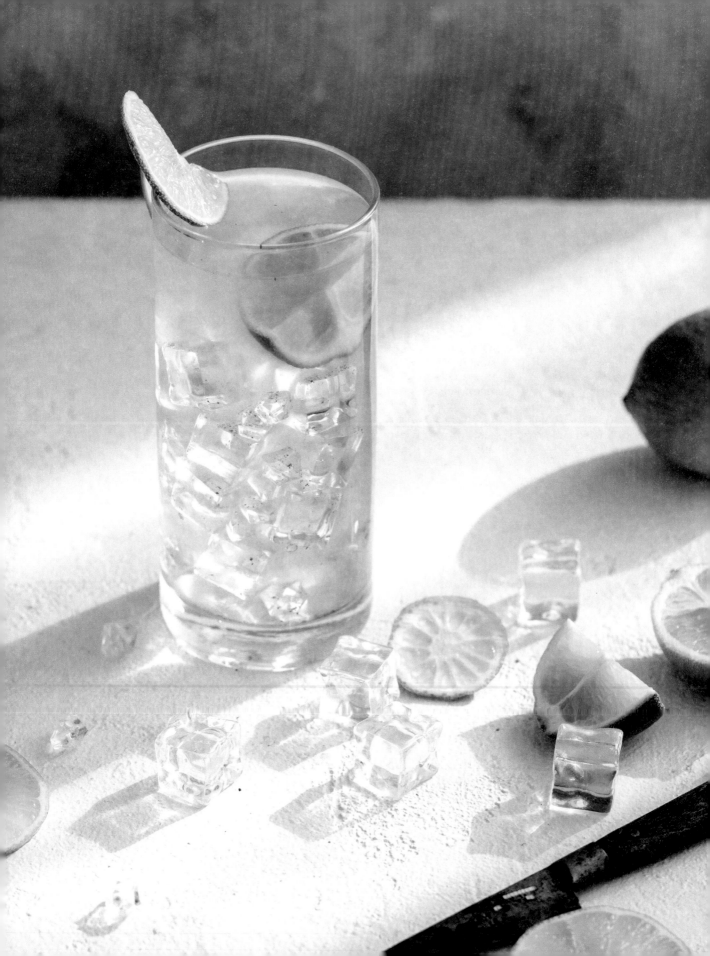

# Keto Kocktail

Most people are now aware of the idea of "ketosis," a metabolic state that occurs when your body burns fat instead of glucose for energy. A keto diet—which is typically low in carbohydrates and high in fat—has many benefits, including potential for greater weight loss, increased energy, better focus, enhanced physical endurance, and managing conditions such as obesity, diabetes, and liver disease.

However, what many people are not aware of is that the same drinkable ketones that have been used for years by biohackers, athletes, and even the military for enhanced performance with limited calories and carbohydrates can also be used—drumroll, please—as a healthy, effective, and surprisingly pleasant substitute for an evening cocktail or serving of alcohol, without any of the potentially toxic or liver-stressing breakdown products of alcohol. (Don't get me wrong; I have nothing against a glass of organic wine or a healthy cocktail, but it's nice to have an alternative for when you don't want to drink alcohol or need a bit of a detox.)

One form of drinkable ketones, with the sexy name R-1,3 Butanediol, is now emerging as a popular alcohol alternative for social confidence, relaxation, boosting mood, and crushing appetite. I've started experimenting with these ketones for an evening beverage by mixing them with ingredients such as artisanal vinegars, electrolytes, and stevia, and couldn't help but share one of those recipes here.

1. Put the ketones, electrolytes, and apple cider vinegar in a cocktail shaker with ice and shake for 10 to 30 seconds.

2. Pour over a glass of tonic water.

3. Garnish with the lemon wedge.

*Yield:* 1 SERVING

*Total Time:* 5 MINUTES

**TOOLS AND MATERIALS**

Cocktail shaker

**INGREDIENTS**

1 serving liquid ketones

1 packet flavored electrolytes

½ ounce apple cider vinegar

Tonic water, sparkling water, and/or ice

Lemon or lime wedge

***Note:*** *For liquid ketones, I recommend HVMN's Ketone-IQ or KetoneAid Ke4. Incidentally, KetoneAid also has a variety of done-for-you canned ketone cocktails, with flavors such as Moscow Mule, Gin & Tonic, and Piña Colada. For electrolytes, I recommend Protekt watermelon or LMNT citrus salt flavors.*

## A KETONE WARNING

A quick warning: I don't recommend mixing ketones with alcohol. There can be some metabolic tomfoolery that takes place and results in excessive sleepiness, grogginess, and lethargy that aren't very convenient, unless, I suppose, you really want to crash out for the night.

# Cacao Charcoal Latte

You've no doubt seen trendy, black activated charcoal drinks at a local juicery, or noticed activated charcoal capsules being recommended for detoxification or as a popular hangover remedy. Or as an addition to a first aid kit for digestive issues, food poisoning, or even to sop up accumulated metals after a big sushi feed (not a bad idea, really).

If you want to use activated charcoal for any of the reasons listed above, or just want a creamy, frothy, chocolate detox drink with a unique color twist, you should consider using activated charcoal powder or broken-open activated charcoal capsules in a latte recipe like this one.

By the way, charcoal is so effective at soaking stuff up that I wouldn't pair this latte with any vitamins or medications, because you'll be unlikely to absorb much of anything you consume along with the charcoal.

1. Warm the milk in a pot or saucepan. Add the charcoal, sweetener, cacao powder, and salt and whisk until combined.

2. Pour into a mug and use a frothing wand to blend until frothy.

*Yield:* 1 SERVING

*Total Time:* 5 MINUTES

**TOOLS AND MATERIALS**

Pot or saucepan

Whisk

Frothing wand

**INGREDIENTS**

1 cup milk of choice

2 to 4 activated charcoal pills, or about 1 teaspoon charcoal powder

Sweetener of choice, to taste

1 tablespoon organic cacao powder

Pinch of salt

**Note:** *For sweetener, I recommend a dropperful of Omica Organics vanilla.*

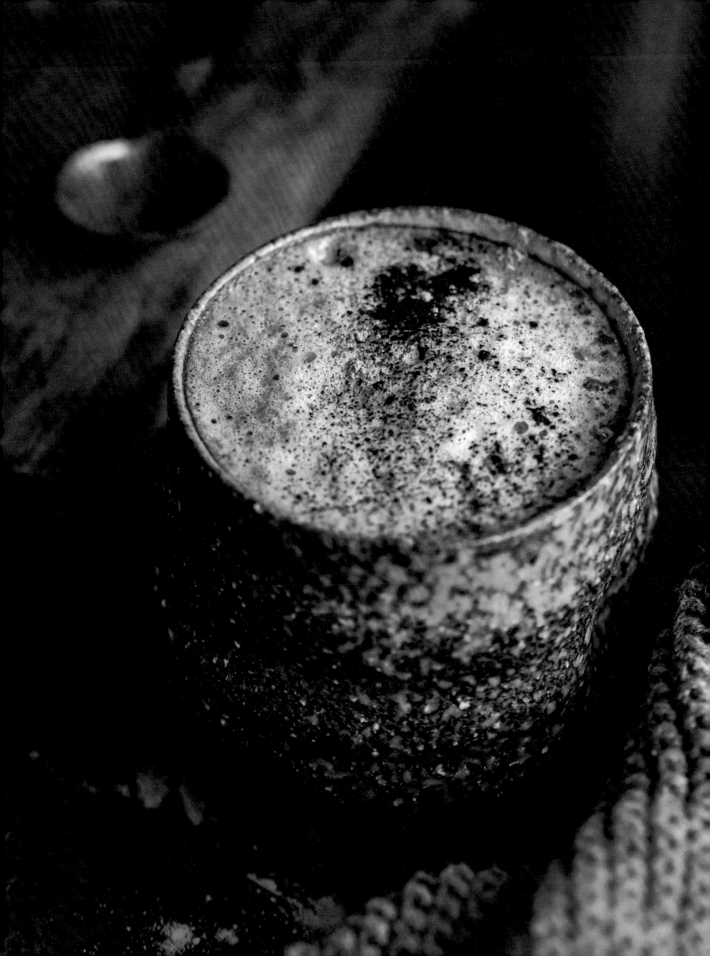

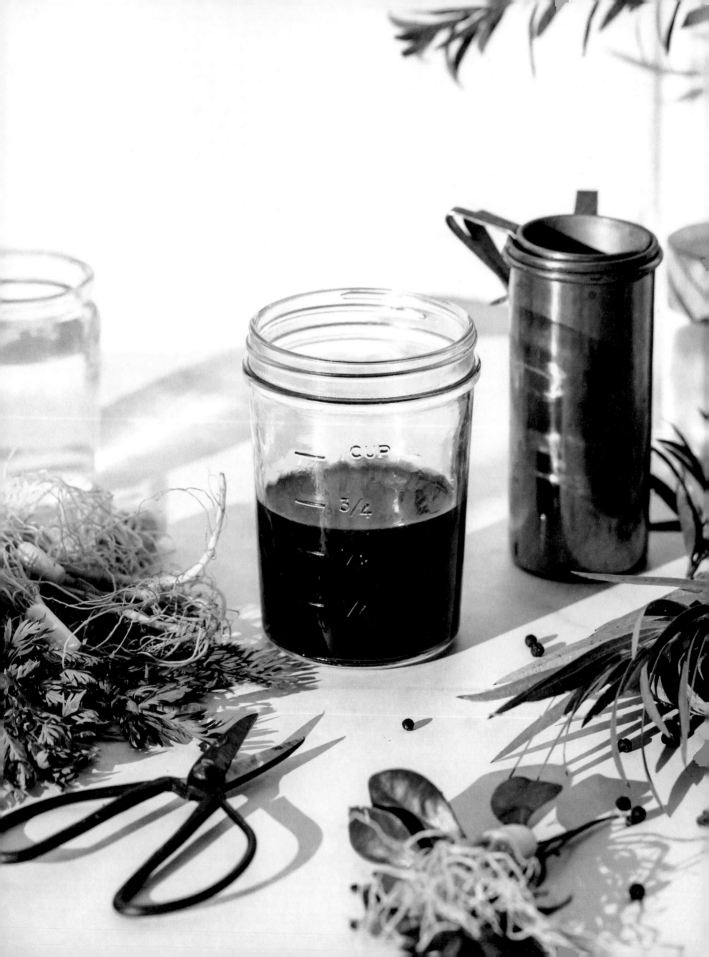

# Backyard Bitters

Certain compounds known as blood glucose disposal agents (BDAs, baby), when consumed prior to eating or drinking, help lower the blood sugar response to a carbohydrate-rich meal or beverage. Many of these same agents can spark the production of enzymes and hormones that help ease digestion, reduce post-meal sluggishness, and increase nutrient absorption.

   This is why in many cultures the consumption of a so-called "digestif" or "aperitif" is a common and traditional practice before, during, or after a meal. In the spirit of connecting with nature, foraging, and digging around in your own backyard for nifty things to eat or drink, I recently came up with this backyard bitters recipe that is a great addition to sparkling water on ice, can be used to temper the sweetness of any random cocktail, or even just serves as something you can drip straight into your mouth should you find yourself wanting a bit of enzymatic help to digest a meal. Yes, it does have trace amounts of alcohol, since that's what's used to extract the goodness from the plants, but it's a trace. Pay close attention to the ratios in this recipe. They're important if you want a decent final product.

1. Combine the alcohol, bitters, and berries in a glass jar, covering the solid ingredients with the liquid.

2. Cover the jar and let it sit for two weeks in a dark place, like the corner of your pantry, giving the jar a shake once or twice a day.

3. Strain off the solids using a fine mesh strainer.

4. In a measuring cup, measure how many ounces of alcohol you have left after straining and then set that alcohol aside. You'll need it later, so don't toss it.

5. Measure out twice as much water as alcohol, put the water into a small saucepan, add the strained solids, and bring the mixture to a boil.

6. Reduce the heat and simmer for about 10 minutes.

7. Remove the water and solids from the heat, add the mixture to a jar or other container, cover it, and let it sit for 12 to 24 hours.

8. Strain out the solids and discard them.

9. Measure how much liquid is left, pour it into a saucepan, and add 1 teaspoon of sugar for every four ounces of liquid. Warm this liquid on low to medium heat while you whisk to dissolve the sugar. Then remove it from the heat and allow the liquid to cool.

10. Combine this cooled, water-based liquid with the alcohol liquid. Boom: you've now got bitters.

11. Transfer the bitters to dropper or spritzer bottles, and use in any creative way you desire with cocktails, mocktails, soda water, or even smoothies.

*Yield:* APPROXIMATELY 6 OUNCES

*Total Time:* APPROXIMATELY 20 MINUTES OF PREPARATION TIME, APPROXIMATELY 2 WEEKS OF WAITING TIME, PLUS AN ADDITIONAL 24 HOURS OF WAITING TIME AFTER STRAINING

## TOOLS AND MATERIALS

Two glass jars

Fine mesh strainer

Measuring cup

Small saucepan

Small dropper bottles or spritzer bottles

## INGREDIENTS

Approximately 4 ounces strong alcohol with neutral flavor, such as Everclear 151

Approximately 1 ounce (if you want to use a small kitchen scale, that's about 30 grams) dried, chopped backyard bitters

Approximately 1 ounce dried, crushed berries (I use Oregon grape berries from my backyard, but other options include blueberries, raspberries, or blackberries)

Sugar, per ratio described below

***Notes:*** *Regarding backyard bitters, dandelion root is easy to find, but mugwort root, Oregon grape root, burdock root, yellow dock root, and chicory root also grow in many backyards. If you're lazy or afraid of the outdoors, you can also buy bitter roots from places like OldTownSpiceShop.com or even Amazon, but what fun is that?*

*If you like this recipe, you may also want to check out the book* The Wildcrafted Cocktail, *which holds a hallowed place in my kitchen for when I want to go out like a dirty hippie in nature to find my drinks instead of getting all dressed up and venturing to a fancy martini bar.*

# Immune-Boosting Elderberry Syrup

*The following recipe is a contribution from my friend and manager of the Ben Greenfield Life coaching program, Sarah Frazier.*

I first learned the power of elder a few years ago while diving into homeopathic health concepts. I had injured myself and was looking for healing via every natural method possible. In my research I discovered homeopathic remedies for insomnia, anxiety, headaches, and immunity, but something called elder kept coming up as one of the best go-tos for overall immune health. Elder is a genus of flowering plants that look more like a giant bush-shaped, thick tree, with various species commonly referred to as elder, elderflower, or elderberry.

Compounds found particularly in elderberry block some of the sites that viruses use to get into your cells, helping keep your immune system at peak performance. Elderberries are also loaded with antioxidants, thanks to their deep blue-purple pigments. Meanwhile, elderflower—the flowering component of the elder plant—acts as an antihistamine that can relieve cold, flu, and even allergy symptoms, and foster a healthy fever response. Components of the elder plant are extremely safe and are often used for adults, children, and the elderly alike for daily immune health, as well as for a boost when you are feeling under the weather.

For this elderberry syrup, I also choose to add raw local honey to increase the allergy-fighting benefits of honey produced by the bees that pollinate my local environment.

1. In a heat-safe glass bowl or measuring cup, combine the elderberries, elderflower, ginger, and cinnamon.

2. Pour the boiling water over the plants. Add the vodka and mix to allow the water and vodka to seep into the plants.

3. Cover with a tea towel or cheesecloth and let the mixture steep for at least 8 hours. I usually mix this in the evening and let it sit overnight.

4. After steeping, use a cheesecloth or a fine mesh strainer to strain the liquid from the herbs into another glass measuring cup. Squeeze as much liquid out as you can and discard the plants.

5. To the strained mixture, add the lemon juice.

6. Measure how much liquid you have. Add equal parts honey to the mixture, a 1:1 ratio. Mix well until the honey is fully dissolved and no longer settles at the bottom.

7. Store the syrup in an amber glass bottle in a room-temperature cabinet.

*Yield:* APPROXIMATELY 6 OUNCES

*Total Time:* 5 MINUTES TO MIX INGREDIENTS; 8 HOURS TO STEEP; 5 MINUTES TO STRAIN, MIX HONEY, AND STORE

## TOOLS AND MATERIALS

Glass bowl or measuring cup

Cheesecloth or fine mesh strainer

Amber glass bottle for storage

## INGREDIENTS

¼ cup dried elderberries

2 tablespoons dried elderflowers

2 teaspoons sliced ginger, not peeled

½ cinnamon stick, crushed

4 ounces boiling water

2 ounces 100-proof vodka (this is for shelf stability; for fridge stability, you can use 1 ounce of 80-proof vodka instead)

Juice of ½ lemon

Raw local honey

**Note:** *Recommended dosage is 1 to 2 teaspoons whenever you want a big immune boost. Per day all winter season, I recommend ½ teaspoon, which you can actually take hourly if you are ill.*

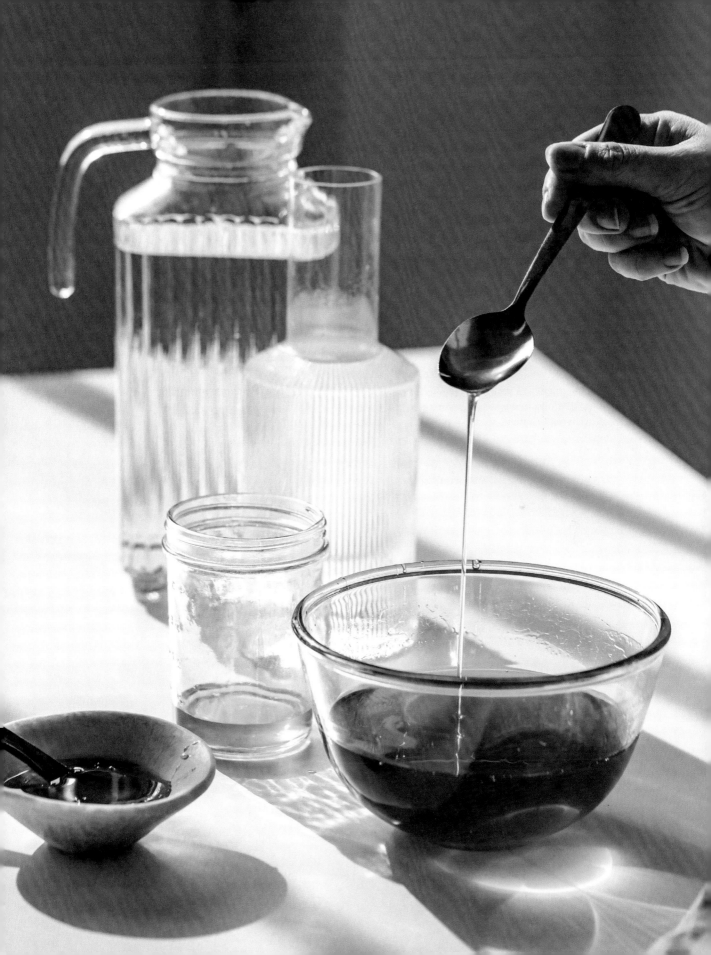

# Smoothies

When I was 15 years old, one of my side gigs was working at my parents' drive-through coffee stand in Moscow, Idaho. While I certainly savored the process of making latte art in the foamy milk atop coffee drinks, suggesting to customers new flavor combinations I'd stumbled upon (such as a pumpkin-spice-vanilla-marshmallow mocha specialty), and eating far too many of the day-old baked goodies at the end of my work shift, one of my favorite parts of the job was manning the ol' blender.

*For all resources, books, tools, and ingredients mentioned throughout this chapter, go to: BoundlessKitchen.com/resources*

Like many coffee shops and stands, ours was equipped with one of those mighty, powerful blenders and blades that could pulverize just about anything you dropped in. So, although up until that point I was a standard bacon 'n' eggs breakfast guy, I began experimenting with drinking smoothies in the morning and inventing new smoothie recipes to add to the ever-expanding drive-through menu.

One of my favorite times of year was when fresh strawberries were in season. This particular coffee stand was located inside a natural foods and produce store, and each spring, when oodles of giant, sweet strawberries from local farms arrived at the produce stand, several buckets of berries would find their way into the mini freezer under the espresso machine. During these times of ripe produce season, I'd spend the downtime between customers inventing, blending, and tasting everything from strawberry-banana-butter-lettuce to dark-chocolate-strawberry-walnut-butter to peppermint-lavender-strawberry-cilantro smoothies (yep, that last one was a total fail). Later, when I began working at my parents' larger coffee shop/pub downtown, I became famous for

blending fruit-forward cabernet and merlot wines with ice, berries, and different syrupy fruit flavors to make a sort of frozen, blended, daiquiri-esque sangria, which, looking back, I now consider a total bastardization of a good wine. (But at the time, I was pretty darn proud of myself for inventing one of the most popular drinks on the nighttime beverage list.)

Fast forward 25 years, and I'm still "that smoothie guy." Not only do I have some kind of a superfood smoothie for breakfast nearly every morning of the week, but when friends visit and stay overnight in our guesthouse, I'll often invite them in to try their first raw liver smoothie, promising that my version tastes just like chocolate ice cream (it really does—check out the Liver Lifeblood Smoothie recipe on page 105). I would whip up colostrum-blueberry blends with fresh homemade yogurt and blend avocado, cacao, vanilla, stevia, sea salt, and coconut butter for scrumptious, guilt-free desserts. So of course I'd be remiss to not include a few of my favorite smoothie recipes here, with the hope that you will learn to burn through blender engines just as fast as I can.

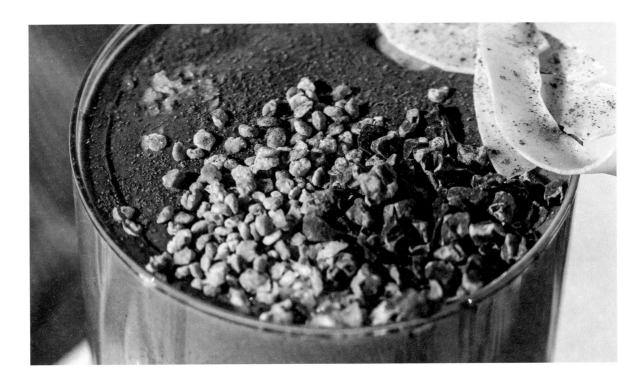

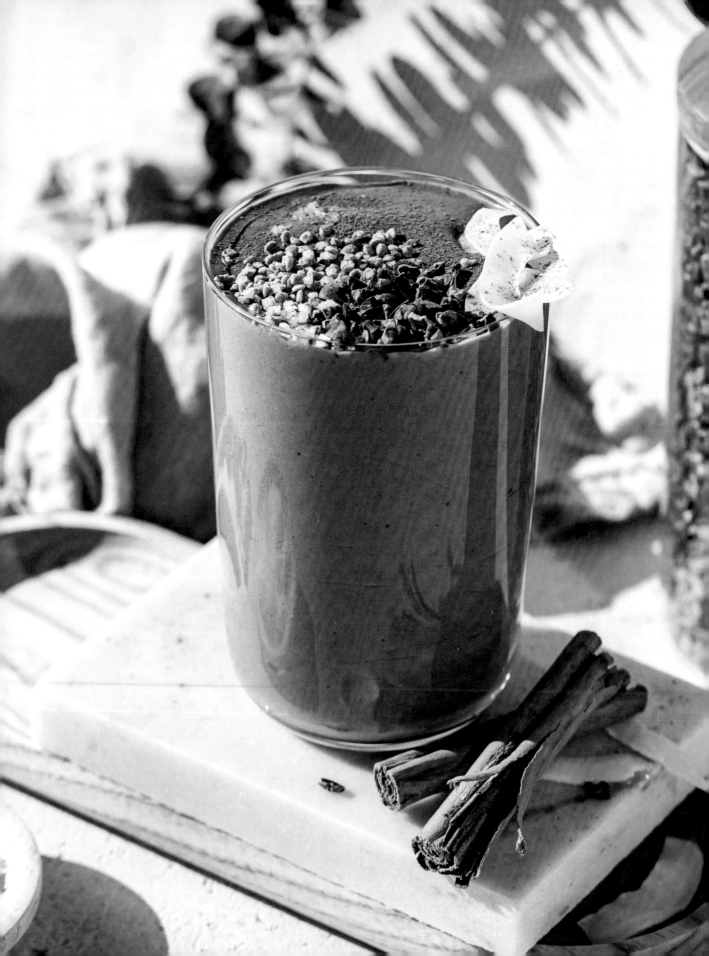

# Liver Lifeblood Smoothie

*"This tastes just like chocolate ice cream!"* That is the most common explanation I get from any of my brave friends to whom I offer a spoonful of my now mildly famous raw liver morning smoothie. Most of them then proceed to beg me for the recipe. I know, I know: it *sounds* disgusting, but I've figured out how to make liver, consumed in the form of a nourishing morning smoothie, actually taste like chocolate ice cream. And furthermore, within 20 minutes after consuming this smoothie, you will feel a surge of clean, pure, unparalleled energy surging through your bloodstream, hence the term *lifeblood*.

If you've been paying attention to the hype in all the ancestral living and eating circles, you know that liver is really, really good for your overall biology. For example, it is the highest source in nature of bioavailable vitamin A in the form of retinol. Unlike vegetables such as carrots, which are rich in carotene, the retinol in liver doesn't need to go through any extra conversion rates to make it highly bioavailable. This high vitamin A content can help with hormone balance and thyroid function, while also playing a key role in liver health and detoxification. In addition, many traditional cultures consider liver to be a "sacred" food, well known for its full-body revitalizing properties and even used to promote fertility. In many ancestral diets, eating liver on a regular basis was encouraged for any couples trying to conceive. Interestingly, liver also contains a yet-to-be-identified "anti-fatigue factor." In one well-known animal study, liver consumption prevented rats that had been swimming for two straight hours from experiencing exhaustion, most likely due to liver's support for the adrenal glands.

1. Soak the liver in the buttermilk for 24 hours in a glass jar or other container.

2. Strain out the soaking liquid, rinse the liver, and blend it in a blender until it is fully puréed.

3. Pour the purée into silicone molds and freeze it for 2 weeks (you can transfer it to a Ziploc bag or other container after 24 hours so it doesn't get freezer burn).

4. Mix the remaining ingredients except toppings in a blender with 2 to 4 small chunks of frozen liver (about 1 to 2 ounces of liver).

5. Blend until it's nice and thick, the consistency of chocolate ice cream.

6. Pour it into a large bowl, mug, or glass and add all the toppings of your choice.

7. Mow down with a spoon and enjoy.

*Yield:* 1 TO 2 SERVINGS

*Total Time:* 24-HOUR SOAK, 2 WEEKS TO FREEZE YOUR LIVER BATCH, AND THEN 5 MINUTES TO MAKE YOUR SMOOTHIE

## TOOLS AND MATERIALS

Glass jar or other container

Blender

Small silicone freezer molds

## INGREDIENTS

1 to 2 pounds fresh liver

Buttermilk or kefir, enough to soak the liver

Bone broth or coconut milk to desired texture (I like enough to blend my smoothie thick like ice cream)

Ice to desired texture (typically about twice as much ice as liquid works well)

1 teaspoon salt

1 teaspoon cinnamon

Stevia, to taste

Chocolate whey protein powder

Toppings: cacao nibs and/or bee pollen and/or coconut flakes or shredded coconut, or a frozen Kion Clean Energy Bar chopped into chunks

1 to 2 heaping tablespoons Gut-Healing Super Yogurt (optional: see page 75)

**Note:** *I use the Reese's Peanut Butter cup–size silicone molds from Amazon—so don't come over to my house and eat the frozen "peanut butter cups" or you'll be in for a surprise. For stevia in this recipe, I recommend Omica Organics vanilla. For the protein whey powder, Kion Clean Protein is delicious!*

# Blueberry–Colostrum Kion Superfood Smoothie

While it may sound mysterious, colostrum probably isn't new to you. In fact, it was likely the first food you ever had. Colostrum is a natural, milky fluid produced by mammals as the first source of nutrition for their young. Science has now shown that it promotes total body health by enhancing immune function, gut health, and athletic recovery.

Colostrum contains a host of natural sources of vitamins, minerals, proteins, and enzymes such as: Cytokines, which are messengers that keep the channels of communication open between the cells in your immune system; lactoferrin, an important protein that supports the health of the intestinal lining and plays a role in the immune system; immunoglobulins (IgA, IgD, IgE, IgG, IgM), which function as antibodies that mediate the body's immune response; proline-rich polypeptides (PRPs), amino acids that help regulate the immune system and support the production of white blood cells; and growth factors (IGF-I, IGF-II, EGF), which are essential hormones that help build and maintain tissues in your GI tract.

Obviously, colostrum has a lot going for it. So, why not *combine* colostrum with another of nature's top superfoods: blueberries? Blueberries are a health and age-reversal powerhouse. They can help cardiovascular performance, bone strength, skin quality, blood pressure, diabetes management, cancer prevention, and mental health, and when paired with animal-based proteins, increase the mobility and density of stem cells.

Now, if you're super focused on a healthy diet and body composition, you may wonder if all those blueberries in a morning smoothie will pack too large a blood sugar punch. While it's true that I generally don't eat carbohydrates until the very end of the day, I'm a huge fan of this smoothie during the summer because heat and sunlight exposure tend to make you more insulin-sensitive. Furthermore, I often make an exception for low glycemic index berries such as blueberries, which cause far less of a blood sugar spike than larger fruits such as melons, apples, and pears.

This superfood smoothie *also* incorporates whey protein from grass-fed, pasture-raised cows that are antibiotic-free and growth hormone–free; creatine for science-backed longevity, muscle, and mental performance; and frozen, crunchy chocolate-nut bars for a guilt-free topping. The smoothie is creamy, delicious, low-calorie (especially if you use bone broth or unsweetened almond or oat milk instead of coconut milk), and incredibly nourishing for every last cell in your body.

1. Blend the first six ingredients until your smoothie reaches the creamy, smooth consistency of ice cream.

2. Top with the energy bar chunks and enjoy.

---

*Yield:* 1 TO 2 SERVINGS

*Total Time:* 3 MINUTES

**TOOLS AND MATERIALS**

Blender

**INGREDIENTS**

½ cup frozen organic blueberries

1 scoop Kion Clean Protein (vanilla or unflavored are best in this recipe)

2 scoops Kion Colostrum

1 scoop Kion Creatine

Coconut milk, unsweetened almond or oat milk, or bone broth to desired texture (usually 4 to 8 ounces)

Ice to desired texture

½ frozen Kion Clean Energy Bar, chopped

**Note:** *Definitely choose organic when purchasing blueberries because these can carry a surprising amount of pesticides. Kion Colostrum is my preferred brand, as it is also from grass-fed, pasture-raised cows, of a single-origin, non-GMO, and contains no antibiotics or hormones. The Kion Clean Energy Bar is delicious, chocolate-nutty goodness and is way better than cacao nibs or nuts.*

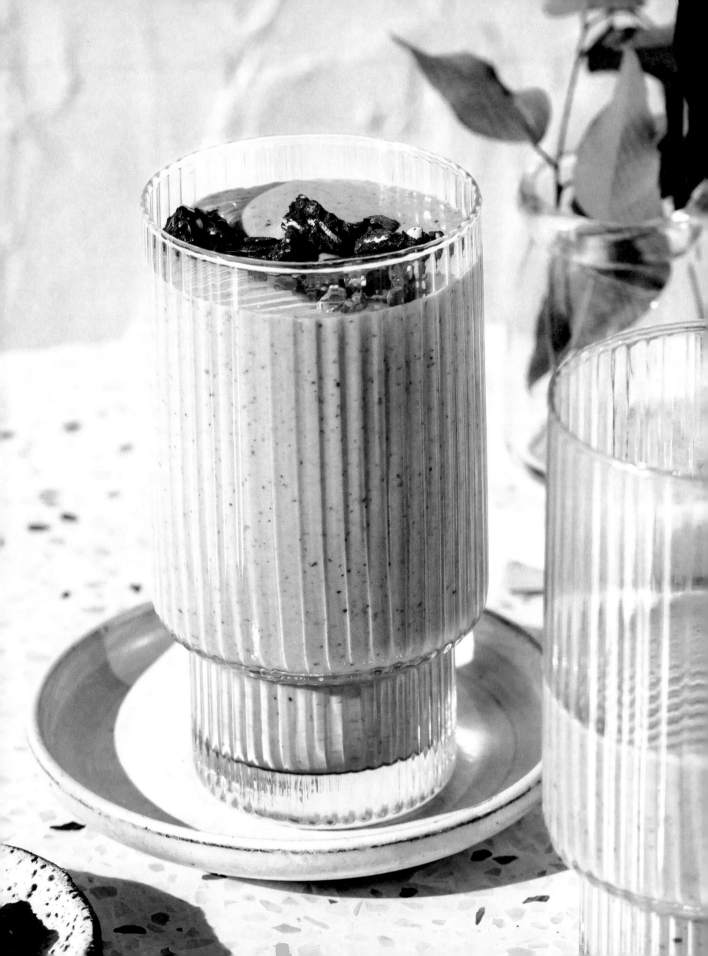

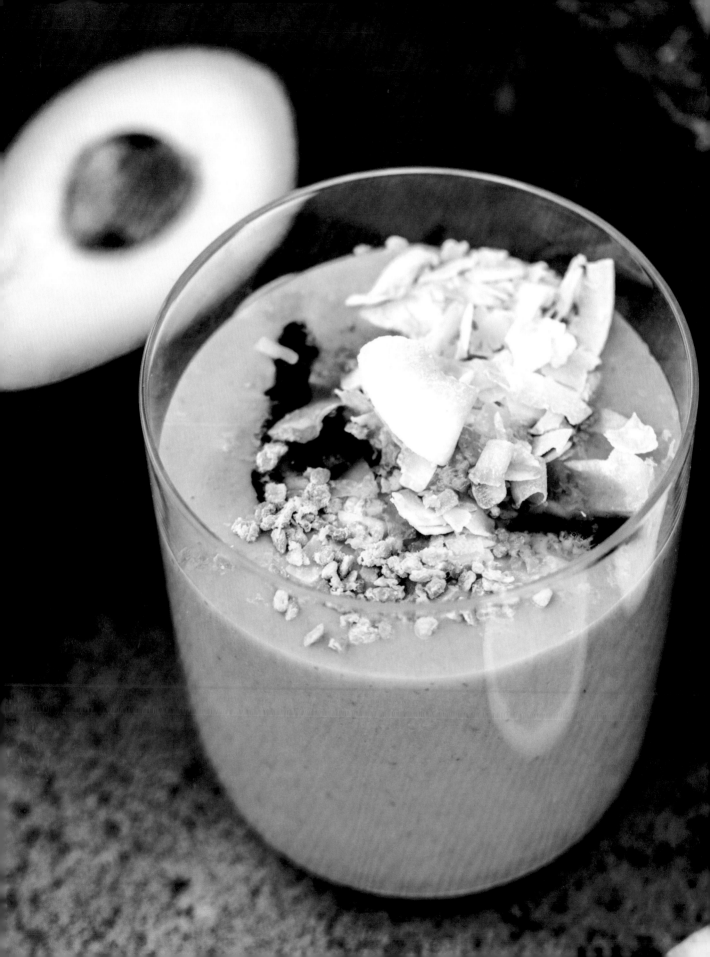

# Citrus Avocado Smoothie

*Yield:* 1 TO 2 SERVINGS

*Total Time:* 2 TO 3 MINUTES

**TOOLS AND MATERIALS**

Blender

**INGREDIENTS**

½ to 1 whole frozen avocado (see freezing instructions on this page), depending on how hungry you are

1 tablespoon broken-up or powdered/pulverized avocado pit (optional)

Juice of 1 lemon or lime plus the zest (zest is optional)

¼ cup coconut milk

1 teaspoon vanilla extract

1 teaspoon maple syrup or honey (or alternative calorie-free sweetener of your choice)

Ice to desired texture

Unsweetened coconut flakes or coconut shreds for a topping

Bee pollen for a topping (optional)

**Note:** *If you choose to add bee pollen, Beekeeper's Naturals has really tasty pollen, and it's wonderful as a smoothie topping.*

Fear not. Avocado smoothies do *not* taste like cold guacamole. Avocados are a handy source of vitamins C, E, K, and $B_6$; high in nutrients like riboflavin, niacin, folate, pantothenic acid, magnesium, potassium, lutein, and beta carotene; and chock-full of omega-3 fatty acids and fats in general, which increases satiety and adds a creamy texture to any smoothie.

To blend or not to blend the pit, also known as the seed, is up to you. Avocado pits actually have more antioxidants than many fruits and vegetables; contain as many polyphenols as green tea; and are full of soluble fiber, phosphorus, potassium, calcium, magnesium, nitrogen, and more. Yes, you may burn through your blender engine and blades more quickly if you make blending the avocado pit a frequent habit, but you can ease the stress on the blender just a bit if you soften the pit first. You can do this by dehydrating the avocado pit in an oven at 250°F for about two hours and then breaking it up with a hammer or blending it all by its lonesome until the pit is pulverized into a powder. You can then add that powder to your smoothies.

Also, it's better to freeze your avocados in advance for a cold, ice cream–like texture (avocados can be frozen for 3 to 6 months and remain well preserved). To do this right, you'll need avocados, lemon juice, plastic wrap, butcher's paper, or beeswax paper, and some airtight containers or bags. First, rinse the avocados, which helps get rid of any dirt on the skin that might transfer inside as you slice them open. You can keep them whole or slice them into halves. Wrap each piece tightly with plastic wrap or beeswax or butcher's paper, place all your wrapped pieces into a freezer bag, and seal the bag tight. If you want to freeze smaller avocado pieces or chunks, just lay them all out on a baking sheet lined with parchment paper or a silicone mat, which flash freezes them, and then remove them from the baking sheet and seal them in freezer bags.

1. Blend together all the ingredients except the toppings to desired consistency.

2. Top with coconut flakes and/or bee pollen, if using.

3. Drizzle with a bit more maple syrup, if desired.

4. Enjoy!

# Keto–Vanilla–Blueberry Bowl

*Yield:* 1 TO 2 SERVINGS

*Total Time:* 2 TO 3 MINUTES

**TOOLS AND MATERIALS**

Blender

**INGREDIENTS**

½ to 1 cup frozen blueberries

Ice to desired texture (about 1 cup)

Full-fat coconut milk to desired texture (about ½ cup)

Stevia, to taste

1 to 2 scoops powdered vanilla-flavored ketones

A pinch of sea salt

Approximately ⅛ of a Keto Brick, chopped into small chunks, flavor of your choice (I recommend Peanut Butter or Milk 'N Cookies.)

**Note:** *I recommend Omica Organics Vanilla Liquid Stevia as well as Perfect Keto Vanilla Flavor for the powdered ketones.*

You've already learned about the magical energy-enhancing, appetite-satiating, anti-inflammatory powers of *liquid* ketones in the Keto Kocktail recipe (see page 95).

But you can also get *powdered* ketones, which act similarly in your body but are handy for something like a smoothie or "acai"-style bowl. Whereas many superfood and acai bowls at the average juicery are north of 600 calories, this easy-to-make bowl has far fewer calories and is very low in carbohydrates.

To stay on-brand with the low-carb approach, I like to top this bowl with a few chopped-up chunks of a Keto Brick. Also featured as a key ingredient of the Fermented Blueberry Cheesecake recipe on page 79, Keto Bricks are one of my favorite sources of on-the-go nutrition, with each "brick" (yes, they're big) packing 1,000 calories, roughly 90 grams of fat, 30 grams of protein, and only 14 grams of total carbs. I bring these with me when I'm hiking or hunting, and if you're an active person who needs massive amounts of low-carb calories for mountaineering, hiking, or hunting, I cannot recommend these enough. They are even shelf-stable above room temperature, which is great for long, hot hiking days.

Besides serving as great fuel for long exertion days, the Keto Brick is also a wonderful topping for any breakfast bowl or smoothie. Just don't eat the whole thing at once (the average topping volume I use for a bowl like the one here is about ⅛ of a brick, chopped into small chunks).

**1.** Place all ingredients except the Keto Brick in a blender and blend as thick as possible, to the consistency of ice cream or thicker.

**2.** Spoon the mixture into a bowl, top with the Keto Brick chunks, and savor with a spoon.

## KETO BRICKS: A LOOK INSIDE

The ingredient profile of a Keto Brick is clean and packed with nutrition. For example, here are the ingredients of the Buttered Maple Pecan flavor: raw organic cacao butter, grass-fed whey protein (maple pecan), pecan butter (roasted pecans), organic Ceylon cinnamon powder, and Himalayan sea salt. Other flavors include ingredients like organic golden flaxseed meal, raw organic fermented cacao nibs, sacha inchi protein, and even ground coffee beans.

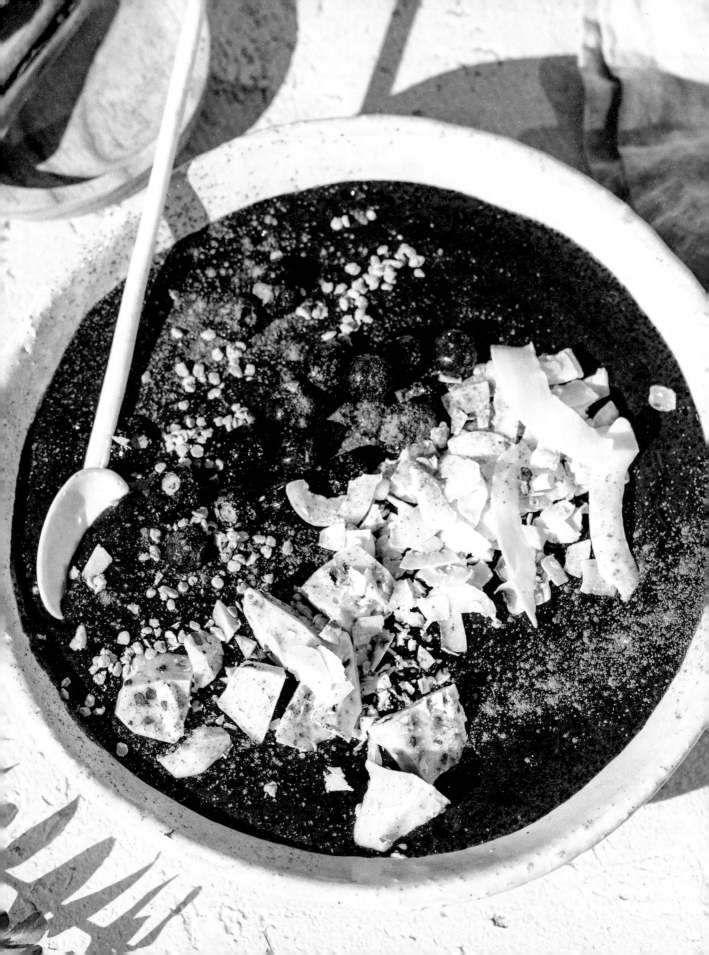

# Desserts

I save nearly all my carbohydrate intake for the evening. It's one of the best "fat loss hacks" I know, and seems to keep energy levels pretty stable too. Basically, if you avoid sugars, starches, sweets, and most other forms of carbs for the majority of the day, you force your body to instead tap into its own storage carbs and fats, especially if you're engaging in activities during the day such as weight training, low-level physical activity, and even cold plunges or cold showers. Think of it like metabolizing a slow-burning log all day long instead of fast-burning kindling.

For all resources, books, tools, and ingredients mentioned throughout this chapter, go to: BoundlessKitchen.com/resources

In the evening I eat as many carbs as I want (within reason) with dinner and/or for dessert, which usually comes out to about 100 to 200 grams of carbs per day. This number of grams per day is still considered to be a low-carb diet, which is a diet that seems to result in pretty stable energy levels for most folks, except, perhaps, professional athletes who exercise for a living—a population that definitely needs more of the fast-burning kindling of carbs.

Perhaps you've heard of the ketogenic diet, which is a very high-fat, very low-carb regimen that allows you to maintain high levels of a stable, long-burning, appetite-satiating, inflammation-reducing energy source called ketones. By saving all your carbs for the evening, you actually get a chance to churn out more of these ketones during the day, produce fewer of them for a brief period of time at night, and then rinse-wash-repeat and begin to churn out ketones again by the following morning. This is technically called a "cyclic ketogenic" diet. I'm not one of those folks who tries to maintain strict ketosis no matter what. My lips zip shut anytime I walk past a bakery or Italian restaurant, and I don't put giant sticks of butter in my tea or keep high-fat coconut butter bombs in the freezer for dessert. But I do appreciate the value of forcing the body to burn its own fat and produce a high amount of ketones for at least some of the day.

This act of consuming carbohydrates primarily in the evening results in a few benefits:

1) evening carbohydrates support the production of serotonin, which can get converted to melatonin, which helps you sleep better; 2) evening carbohydrates—particularly the slow-burning kind such as root vegetables, unprocessed grains, and legumes—keep your energy levels from dipping too low at night, staving off that notorious 1 to 2 A.M. awakening response; and 3) evening carbohydrates top off the body's energy stores for an early-morning workout the next day, which works out quite well for me because I don't like to exercise with a full stomach, so I'm usually doing my morning workout having fasted.

Many nutrition scientists argue that you should instead eat the majority of your carbs in the morning, when your insulin sensitivity is higher due to your cortisol awakening response. While it is indeed true that you are naturally equipped to "handle" carbs better in the morning, you can also skip the carbs and induce a state of temporary insulin sensitivity later in the evening by weight training, walking, swimming, or taking a cold shower at some point in the later afternoon to early evening. Then have your carbs with dinner, allowing you to sort of "have your cake and eat it too"—in this case, quite literally.

These dessert recipes will satisfy your sweet tooth without giving you much of a sugar high or requiring you to make a trip to the grocery store for a pint of tempting yet waistline-expanding ice cream. Enjoy!

# Pumpkin Spice Colostrum Cake

*Yield:* 1 8- OR 9-INCH CAKE

*Total Time:* 1 HOUR, PLUS 4 HOURS FOR REFRIGERATION, IF DESIRED

**TOOLS AND MATERIALS**

Square (8 x 8–inch or 9 x 9–inch) or circular baking dish or circular springform pan (a round cake pan that features a removable bottom and sides)

Parchment paper

Blender

There's nothing quite like a slice of pumpkin spice cake on a crisp fall day. But like most pumpkin spice treats that pop up during the holiday seasons, the average pumpkin-packed baked cake, cookie, or other such treat also tends to be jam-packed with sugar and/or vegetable oils and somewhat lacking in nutrient density. So I decided to take a fall classic and amp up the nutrition quality without sacrificing flavor or texture. Heck, rather than making you feel like you need to take an extra trip to the gym to burn off all the calories and sugar, this treat is actually *good* for nourishing the gut, building muscle, appetite satiation, and much more.

The cake itself contains a host of healthy ingredients, including pumpkin purée, coconut oil, and cardamom, along with two scoops of Kion Clean Protein for building muscle, enhancing recovery, and weight management. The secret ingredient and true nutrition powerhouse in the frosting is of course one of my favorite frosting powerhouses: rich, creamy, gut-nourishing Kion Colostrum.

This recipe makes about one 8- or 9-inch cake. To make a layered cake, you can double the pumpkin spice cake and frosting ingredients. I refrigerate my finished cake for about 4 hours to get it to set to a more solid texture, and when my family and I have eaten our fill, I often hide it away in the freezer to chop up for smoothie toppings and snacks later (shh, don't tell my wife and kids that I hide cake in the dark corners of the freezer).

**INGREDIENTS FOR THE PUMPKIN SPICE CAKE**

One 15-ounce can organic pumpkin purée

3 medium or large eggs

⅓ cup maple syrup

¼ cup coconut oil

1½ teaspoons vanilla extract

1½ teaspoons cinnamon

½ teaspoon nutmeg

½ teaspoon cardamom

¼ teaspoon salt

2 cups almond flour or coconut flour

½ cup arrowroot flour

1 teaspoon baking soda

½ teaspoon baking powder

Two scoops Kion Vanilla Whey Protein

**INSTRUCTIONS FOR THE PUMPKIN SPICE CAKE**

1. Preheat the oven to 350°F. Line the baking dish with parchment paper.

2. In a large bowl, combine pumpkin purée, eggs, maple syrup, coconut oil, vanilla, cinnamon, nutmeg, cardamom, and salt. Mix until smooth.

3. In a separate bowl, whisk together the almond flour, arrowroot, baking soda, baking powder, and whey.

4. Spoon the dry ingredients into the wet ingredients until just combined.

5. Pour the batter into the baking dish and level smooth with a spatula.

6. Bake for 25 to 30 minutes, or until a toothpick inserted in the center comes out clean.

7. Cool on the counter at room temperature or in the refrigerator for around 30 minutes before applying frosting.

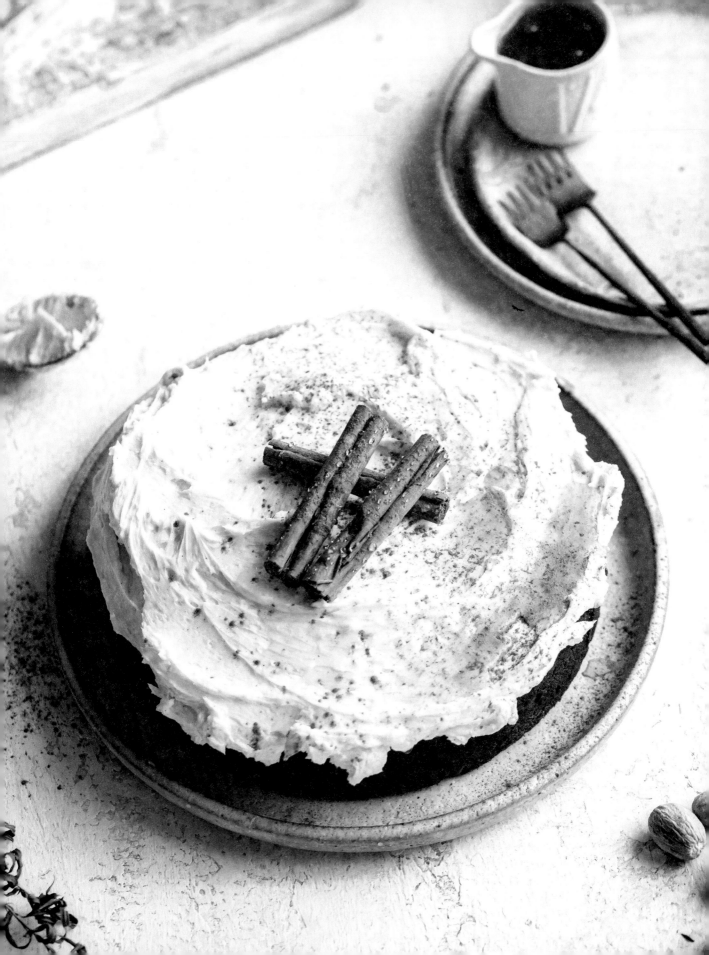

## INSTRUCTIONS FOR THE FROSTING

1. Place the softened butter and cream cheese in a blender and blend until well mixed, about 60 seconds.

2. Add tapioca powder, vanilla extract, colostrum, salt, and stevia.

3. Stir with a whisk or fork until creamy.

4. Spread the frosting generously with a spatula over the cooled cake.

5. Cover with plastic wrap and refrigerate for around 4 hours before slicing and serving.

## INGREDIENTS FOR THE FROSTING

½ cup butter, softened at room temperature

8 ounces cream cheese, room temperature (for dairy-free, use an equivalent amount of coconut cream)

2 cups tapioca powder

2 teaspoons vanilla extract

½ cup Kion Colostrum

⅛ teaspoon salt

Stevia, to taste

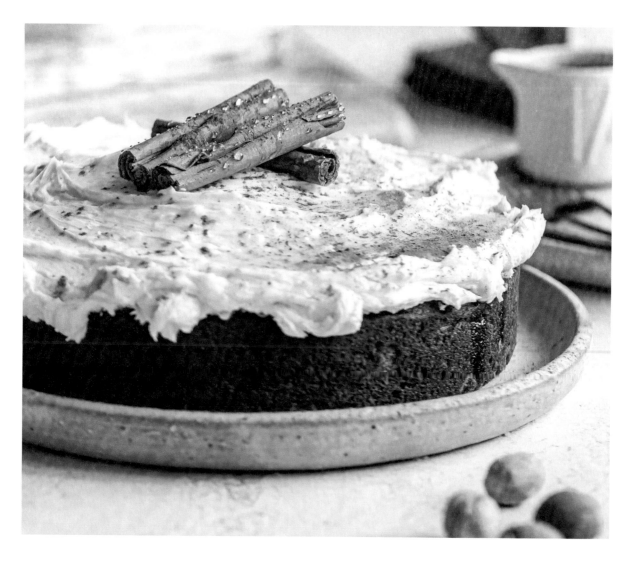

# Purple Carrot Cake

*Yield:* 1 8-INCH CAKE

*Total Time:* 50 MINUTES, PLUS TIME FOR CAKE TO COOL BEFORE FROSTING

## TOOLS AND MATERIALS

8 x 8–inch baking dish

## INGREDIENTS FOR THE CAKE

Avocado oil or olive oil for greasing pan

1 cup almond flour

¾ cup tapioca flour

¼ cup coconut flour

1 teaspoon ground cinnamon

1 teaspoon ground nutmeg

¼ teaspoon ground cloves

½ teaspoon ground ginger

1 teaspoon baking soda

½ teaspoon salt

¼ cup maple syrup

¼ cup honey

1 cup organic pumpkin purée

2 medium or large eggs

½ cup extra-virgin olive oil

1¼ cups shredded purple carrots

1¼ cups chopped walnuts

I'm a big sucker for carrot cake. My entire family is well aware that I have almost no willpower to not overeat it. I almost always eat an extra slice, or two, even if I'm already full. Maybe it's the word *carrot* that makes it seem like I'm eating vegetables, or maybe it's the addicting combination of moist cake with creamy, sweet frosting and a nutty, shredded carrot texture, but I just can't help myself. As a matter of fact, the traditional meal I repeatedly "request" for my birthday and Father's Day is indeed ribeye steak and carrot cake, and it will likely be the last meal I'll request on my deathbed, if I still have teeth and it's an option.

But I'm also an enormous fan of the healthy, cellular root-based carbohydrate pumpkin, including in the form of baked pumpkin slices drizzled with raw honey and sprinkled with coarse salt and cinnamon; organic pumpkin purée blended with yogurt and dark chocolate for dessert; foamy pumpkin spice lattes sprinkled with cinnamon; and, of course, massive amounts of pumpkin flavor infused into my favorite dessert: carrot cake. It's a match made in heaven.

And as for the purple? While all carrots, independent of their color, are packed with a variety of nutrients, such as fiber, potassium, vitamin C, manganese, vitamin A, and B vitamins, what makes purple carrots unique is their rich content of anthocyanins. Anthocyanins belong to the polyphenol family of antioxidants and are found in purple fruits and vegetables like blackberries, grapes, purple potatoes, purple cabbage, and purple carrots. They help protect your body from oxidative stress, which is an imbalance between reactive molecules called free radicals and antioxidants in your body, and they are particularly helpful for staving off heart disease, mental decline, and diabetes. And let's face it: orange is just way too traditional for a biohacked cookbook, right? You should be able to find purple carrots at most grocery stores or farmers markets, and it's pretty simple to grow your own too. Hint: this recipe works fine with regular carrots too.

## INSTRUCTIONS FOR THE CAKE

1. Preheat the oven to 350°F. Grease an 8 x 8–inch baking dish with avocado oil (it can be handy to have avocado oil spray on hand for this).

2. In a large bowl, mix together the almond flour, tapioca flour, coconut flour, cinnamon, nutmeg, cloves, ginger, baking soda, and salt.

3. In another large bowl, whisk together the maple syrup, honey, pumpkin purée, eggs, olive oil, and 1/4 cup water until the mixture thickens to a batter-like consistency.

4. Pour the bowl of dry ingredients into the bowl of wet ingredients and mix well.

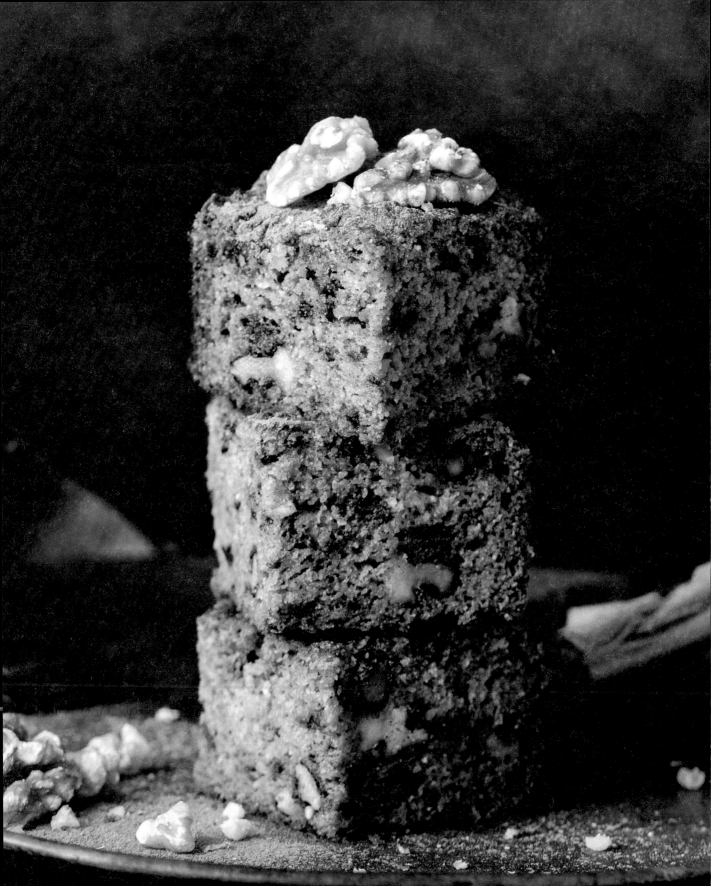

5. Fold the shredded carrots and chopped walnuts thoroughly into the batter.

6. Pour the batter into the greased pan and smooth the top with a spatula.

7. Bake for 35 to 40 minutes, or until a toothpick comes out clean and the surface is slightly golden. Allow the cake to cool for 10 minutes in the pan and then transfer it to a wire rack to cool (preferably in the fridge) to at least room temperature before applying the frosting. Cool for sbout 30 minutes.

## INSTRUCTIONS FOR THE FROSTING

1. While the cake is baking, prepare your frosting. In a small bowl or blender, mix together the almond butter, almond milk, vanilla, maple syrup, cinnamon, and salt until smooth.

2. Drizzle the cake with the frosting, smoothing out with a spatula if desired, and serve.

## INGREDIENTS FOR THE FROSTING

1 tablespoon almond butter

2 tablespoons almond milk

½ teaspoon vanilla

1 teaspoon maple syrup or honey

1 teaspoon cinnamon

1 teaspoon salt

**Note:** *For a lower-calorie frosting option, you can use Omica Organics vanilla- or butterscotch toffee–flavored stevia to taste instead of honey or maple syrup.*

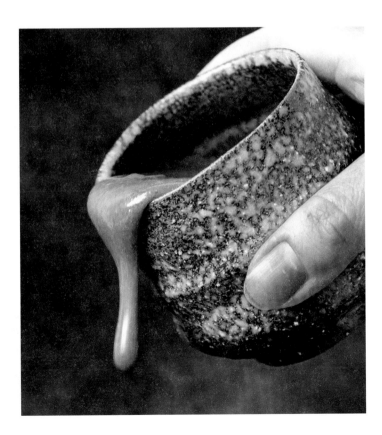

# Barùkas Fudgesicle

*Yield:* 12 POPSICLES

*Total Time:* 10 TO 15 MINUTES TO PREPARE, 5 TO 6 HOURS TO FREEZE

**TOOLS AND MATERIALS**

Blender

Popsicle molds

Parchment paper or waxed paper

**INGREDIENTS**

2 avocados

2 bananas

2 tablespoons honey

2 dropperfuls Omica Organics vanilla stevia

2 teaspoons cinnamon

1 heaping teaspoon salt

2 heaping tablespoons Barùkas nut butter

4 tablespoons organic cacao powder

1 heaping scoop Kion Clean Vanilla Whey Protein (optional, for added health)

One can organic full-fat coconut milk

Barùkas trail mix, for dredging

Every summer we throw an increasingly popular Greenfield summer popsicle party. Everyone arrives in the evening with a cooler containing their own inventive popsicle recipe. Then, after dinner, a few select judges slip away to taste and rank each popsicle based on appearance, flavor, creativity, and overall score. Then all popsicles are unleashed upon a hungry audience armed with butter knives to chop off a piece of each popsicle they want to try. Eventually, the top three popsicles are revealed, and the champion receives some kind of cheesy prize of my choosing.

The variety of popsicle inventions at this party tends to be quite entertaining: from deconstructed ladyfinger, red velvet, and carrot cake popsicles to blueberry crème fraîche to apple pie dipped in crispy crumbles, the sky's the limit. My own contribution? The Barùkas Fudgesicle, which I now share here in all its glory (and yes, you can, if you would like, substitute macadamia nuts, almond nuts, cashews, or other nuts for Barùkas nuts if you have a hard time getting your hands on this addictive, mouthwatering combination of cashew and peanut).

1. Place the avocados, bananas, honey, stevia, cinnamon, salt, Barùkas nut butter, cacao powder, and protein powder, if using, in a blender along with the can of coconut milk. Blend for 2 minutes.

2. After blending, pour the mixture into popsicle molds and freeze them for 5 to 6 hours.

3. Pulverize the Barùkas trail mix in a blender and place it in a separate bowl. Remove the popsicles from the freezer. Then carefully pull the popsicles from their molds one at a time, dip each popsicle into Barùkas nut butter, and dredge them through Barùkas trail mix.

4. Lay each dipped popsicle out on parchment paper placed on a large baking sheet, cover them with plastic wrap, and refreeze them until you're ready to serve.

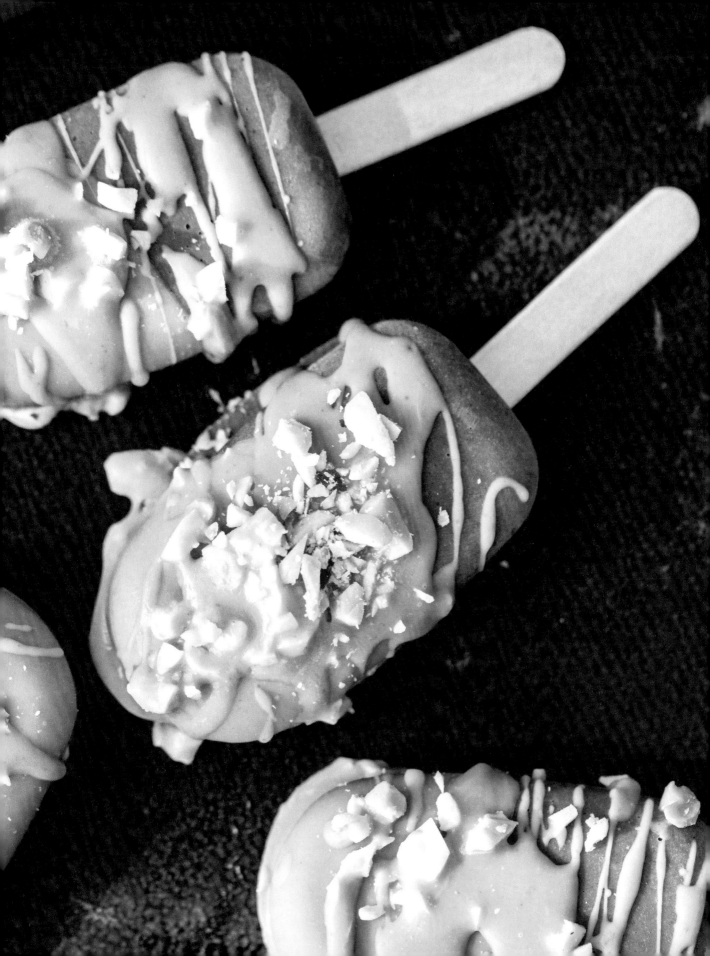

# Baked Blueberry Donuts with Creamy Coconut Glaze

*Yield:* 8 TO 12 DONUTS

*Total Time:* 30 TO 45 MINUTES

**TOOLS AND MATERIALS**

Whisk

Silicone donut molds

**INGREDIENTS FOR THE DONUTS**

1 Serenity Kids Berry Butternut Dairy-Free Smoothie

¼ cup plain yogurt

3 large eggs

2 tablespoons coconut oil, melted and cooled

1 teaspoon vanilla extract

¼ teaspoon apple cider vinegar

1½ cups almond flour

1 cup tapioca flour

2 scoops collagen, unflavored or vanilla

1½ teaspoons baking powder

Pinch of pink Himalayan salt

1 cup fresh organic blueberries

**INGREDIENTS FOR THE COCONUT GLAZE**

¼ cup coconut butter

¼ cup coconut cream

1 teaspoon vanilla extract

1 tablespoon maple syrup or honey (optional) or alternative sweetener of your choice

Unsweetened coconut flakes or bee pollen (optional)

I'm known for eating baby food, often straight from the pouch and squirted into my gaping maw. At other times I use it as a savory salad dressing, a creamy smoothie ingredient, or a low-calorie dessert substitute. But as a grown baby like me should be, I'm quite picky about my baby food, which is why I only eat the stuff from a company called Serenity. You can listen to my podcast with Serenity Carr, the founder of Serenity Baby Foods at BenGreenfieldLife .com/Serenity, but in short, this is the most nourishing, infant-appropriate, and cleanest baby food I've ever discovered. It is jam-packed with tasty, nutrient-dense flavor combinations of pasture-raised meats, organic vegetables, and healthy fats and is designed to neatly match the nutrient ratio properties of breast milk.

These baked blueberry donuts, inspired by Serenity herself, are full of fresh blueberries and topped with a sweet coconut glaze. They're perfect for a weekend breakfast and, if you're like me, even better when dipped into a piping hot mug of black coffee. The primary superstar ingredient in them is, of course, Serenity Kids Dairy-Free Berry Butternut Smoothie (basically a smoothie pouch designed for tots), which contains organic butternut squash, organic coconut cream, organic blueberries, water, organic spinach, hydrolyzed grass-fed bovine collagen, and organic lemon juice.

## INSTRUCTIONS FOR THE DONUTS

1. Preheat the oven to 350°F. Generously spray your donut pan with coconut oil spray. If you're using a silicone donut pan (preferred), you don't need to spray the pan. Set it aside.

2. In a large bowl, whisk together the smoothie pack, yogurt, eggs, coconut oil, and 1 teaspoon of the vanilla extract until a smooth mixture forms.

3. Stir in the apple cider vinegar until just combined.

4. In a separate small bowl, whisk together the almond flour, tapioca flour, collagen, baking powder, and salt until combined.

5. Slowly incorporate the flour mixture into the large bowl with the smoothie mixture ingredients and mix until the batter is smooth and combined.

6. Fold in the blueberries until they are mixed throughout the batter.

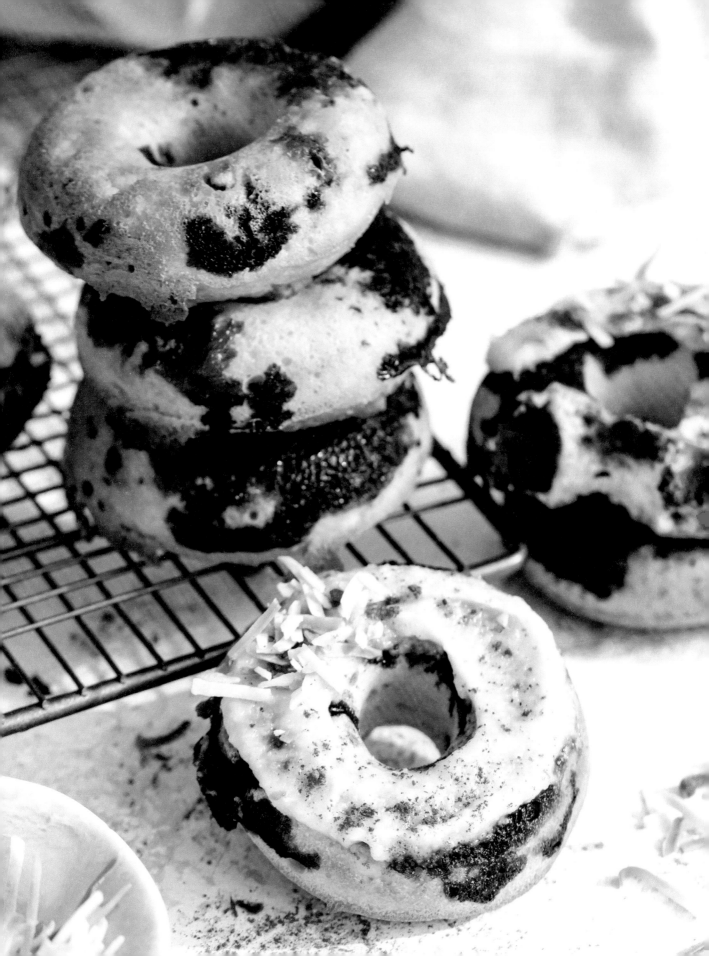

7. Fill each donut mold three-quarters of the way full.

8. Bake for 15 minutes or until a toothpick comes out clean.

9. Allow the donuts to completely cool before popping them out of the mold.

### INSTRUCTIONS FOR THE COCONUT GLAZE

1. In a small saucepan over low heat, whisk together the coconut butter, coconut cream, the remaining 1 teaspoon of vanilla extract, and maple syrup (if using) until mixture is smooth and thick, about 5 to 6 minutes.

### ASSEMBLE THE DONUTS

1. Dunk each donut in the glaze.

2. Sprinkle with unsweetened coconut flakes, if using.

3. Store the donuts in an airtight container in the fridge for up to 4 days.

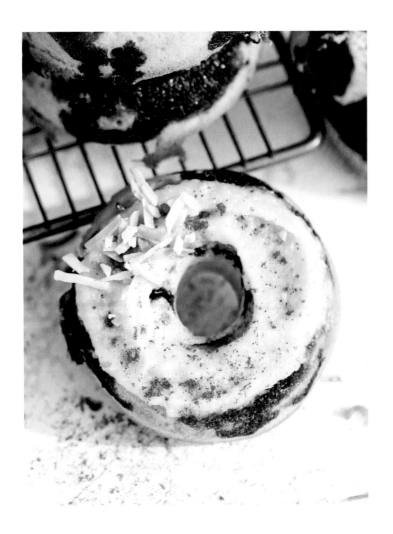

## GUMMIES

While traveling, I recently shopped at a health food store and realized I needed a low-calorie dessert that could manage blood sugar and was similar to the homemade apple cider vinegar gummies I make at home. So I grabbed a tiny jar of so-called ACV gummies, got to the checkout, and realized it was north of 30 bucks for one tiny jar. Fact is, I make them for pennies on the dollar at home.

I've written previously about the host of health benefits in vinegar (see page 89), but when it's combined with gelatin, you've got yourself a tasty powerhouse of a nourishing nutrition bite. Gelatin and collagen are often confused, so allow me to quickly clarify. Collagen is the most abundant form of protein in your body and is composed of amino acids that support your connective tissues, hair, skin, and nails. Gelatin is simply hydrolyzed collagen, meaning that the collagen has been heated to break it down into smaller particles. Furthermore, gelatin makes a gel-like substance when mixed with water, while collagen does not. This gel can help nourish the gut lining and, just like collagen, support healthy hair, skin, and nails. It's also good for your joints and is an easily digestible protein for anyone suffering with gut distress or poor protein digestion.

Because gelatin is made from ground-up dehydrated tendons and ligaments of animals, it does need to be soaked in water or another liquid, such as juice or broth. This softens the gelatin particles so they do not later turn into annoying hardened lumps. Once the gelatin is dissolved, it becomes smooth and translucent and can be easily added to any of your foods. To bloom powdered gelatin, you just sprinkle your desired amount into a pot over any of the cool water or other liquid called for in your recipe and then let the gelatin rest in the liquid for about four minutes.

While the gelatin rests, heat the remaining liquid called for in the recipe to just below a boil. Then gently pour the hot liquid over the gelatin-filled liquid, using a whisk to stir the gelatin crystals completely into the liquid. Ratios are important here: typically, you want about 1.5 teaspoons of gelatin powder to 2 cups of liquid.

Two of my favorite inexpensive, easy-to-make, highly digestible gelatin gummy recipes appear in these pages: Greenfield Turkish Delight (page 131) and Chocolate Chai Gummies (page 132). I keep a big mason jar of these in the refrigerator, although I have to admit I sometimes keep a few in the freezer too and pop them into my mouth like miniature popsicles before or after dinner or lunch. Either also serves as a tasty and unique appetizer for a dinner party.

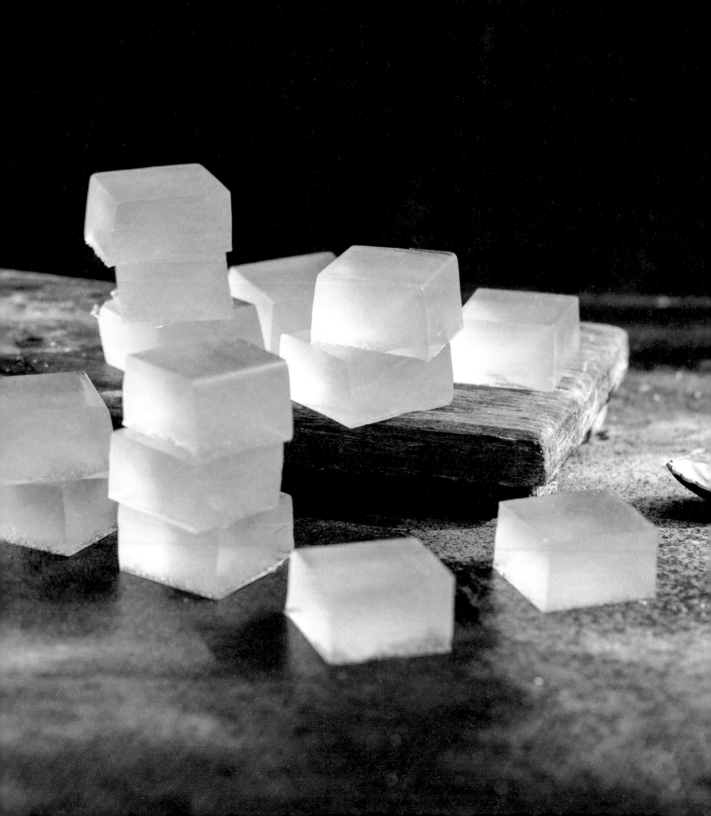

# Deep Sleep Gummies

Considering the sky-high price of most "sleep" gummies on the market, it makes good sense to consider simply making your own—and like other gummy recipes, it's incredibly easy to do. The lecithin in these gummies acts as an emulsifier and stabilizer, allowing oil and water to combine well. This makes it perfect for recipes like these incredibly relaxing deep sleep gummies, which have several different ingredients. Lecithin can also increase the bioavailability of ingredients in a recipe like these gummies, allowing them to be even more potent for pre-sleep use. I recommend popping 2 to 3 gummies about 30 to 45 minutes before bed.

1. Over low to medium heat, stir together the juice, lecithin, honey, and gelatin powder until the gelatin is well dissolved. Let the mixture sit to cool.

2. Stir in 2 to 3 tablespoons of the adaptogen and CBD or other relaxing liquid combo.

3. Pour the gummy mixture into silicone molds.

4. Refrigerate the gummies for at least 4 hours.

*Yield:* 20 TO 30 GUMMIES

*Total Time:* 30 MINUTES TO PREPARE, 4 HOURS TO SET

**TOOLS AND MATERIALS**

Silicone molds

**INSTRUCTIONS**

1 cup organic tart cherry juice

1 teaspoon lecithin (emulsifier)

2 tablespoons honey

4 tablespoons gelatin powder

2 tablespoons adaptogen of choice (see note below), to desired strength

1000 to 5000 milligrams CBD extract, depending on desired gummy strength

2 tablespoons powdered glycine (optional, but helps lower the body's core temperature during sleep!)

**Note:** *For the adaptogen, I recommend liquid or powdered ashwaganda or reishi extract. Alternatively, for a combination of L-theanine and GABA, I use one full bottle of Quicksilver Scientific Liposomal GABA with L-Theanine, which contains 2500 milligrams of L-theanine. For CBD extract, I like Element Health Maximum Strength CBD tincture, which has 4800 milligrams in one bottle— and notably, CBD, unlike THC, will not deleteriously impact deep-sleep cycles or dreaming/memory consolidation.*

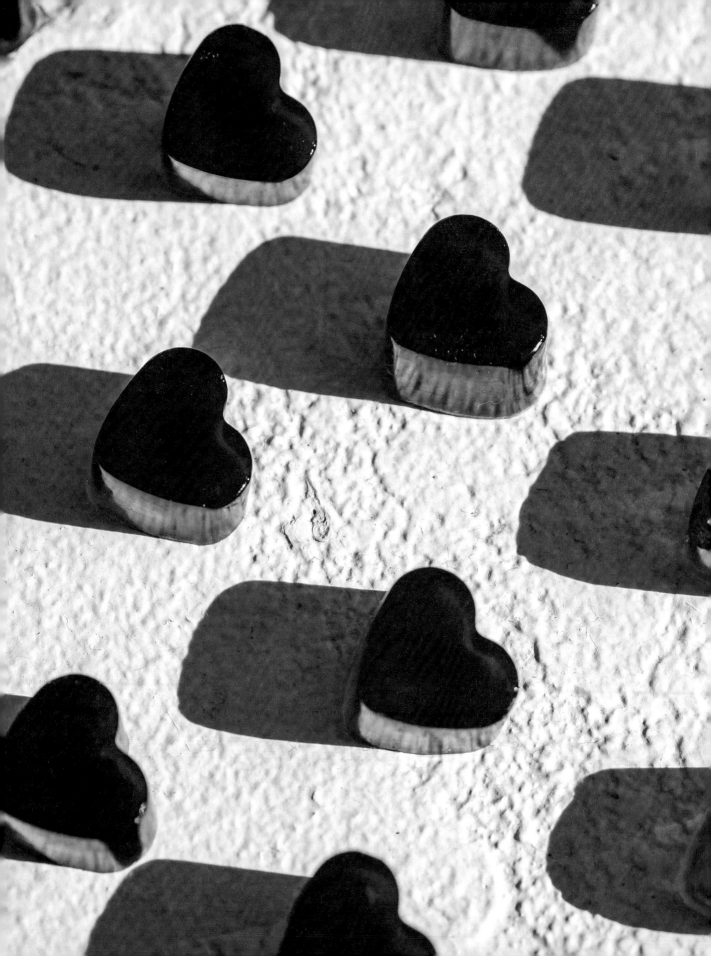

# Amino Jello

My super satiating nighttime jello recipe was one of the most popular "desserts" in the original *Boundless Cookbook*, but the new version here is an enhanced upgrade with the addition of muscle-building and gut-nourishing amino acids and the removal of carbohydrates and sugars.

A few years ago my friends and brilliant biohackers Ron Penna and Joel Greene taught me that gelatin (yes, the same stuff you find in J-E-L-L-O) is a rich source of glycine, an amino acid with a mildly sweet taste that naturally lowers the body temperature pre-sleep and helps your body make serotonin, a hormone and neurotransmitter that has significant effects on sleep and mood, along with a substantial appetite-satiating effect. After that discussion, I began making my own jello for pennies on the dollar (while avoiding the artificial colors and sweeteners of the store-bought stuff) and found it to be an incredibly effective nighttime low-calorie dessert for satiating appetite and improving sleep. I recommend the watermelon or mango flavors for this particular recipe.

1. Pour the juice into a medium-size small saucepan.

2. Sprinkle the gelatin powder over the liquid and stir it in well.

3. Turn the heat on medium-low and bring the liquid to a simmer, stirring occasionally with a fork or whisking until the gelatin is dissolved. This should take 5 to 10 minutes.

4. Turn off the heat and add the allulose, if using.

5. Pour into an 8 × 8–inch square baking dish.

6. Refrigerate until the jello is set, about 2 hours.

*Yield:* 18 TO 20 SERVINGS

*Total Time:* 10 MINUTES PLUS 2 HOURS TO SET

## TOOLS AND MATERIALS

Small saucepan

8 × 8–inch square baking dish

## INGREDIENTS

4 cups fresh fruit juice or coconut water

3 tablespoons grass-fed gelatin powder (add more if you like your jello super firm, which I do)

4 scoops Kion Aminos

2 tablespoons allulose, monk fruit, stevia, or honey (optional)

***Notes:*** *I use coconut water in this recipe but have even experimented with full-fat, organic coconut milk for a bit more creamy and slightly higher-calorie jello.*

*I like to eat about a 2 x 2–inch square before bed. That may seem small, but that's all it seems to take for the potent appetite-satiating and sleep-enhancing effects.*

## THIS JELLO'S SECRET INGREDIENT

The "secret ingredient" in this new jello recipe is Kion Aminos, a blend of essential amino acids (EAAs) that serve as the building blocks of protein, energy, and total body health. They help you grow and maintain lean muscle mass, speed up recovery, improve mental performance, and more. New research shows that EAA supplements rich in the amino acid leucine work even better than traditional EAAs to stimulate muscle protein synthesis, aid in muscle repair, and support athletic recovery. Kion Aminos contain 40 percent leucine, with the remaining EAAs in optimal, scientifically backed ratios shown to help you grow stronger muscles and recover faster.

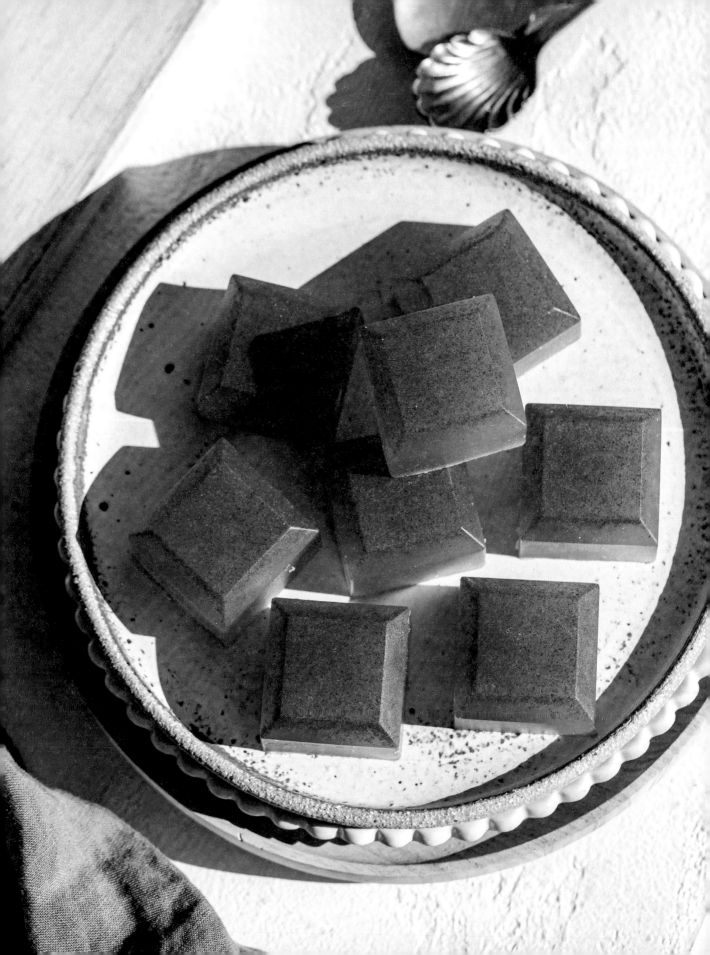

# Greenfield Turkish Delight

Apple cider vinegar provides a whole host of health benefits, from improving insulin sensitivity to lowering post-meal blood glucose, boosting digestion, supporting weight loss, and much more. However, the idea of chugging ACV throughout the day isn't exactly appealing to most folks, and understandably so.

So what is my favorite way to get all the benefits of ACV on a regular basis? Tossing it into some convenient, delicious gummies, of course. I put my own spin on this recipe by swapping out the typical ingredient of raw honey for allulose, which is a low-calorie, zero-sugar sweetener that tends to be easier to digest than most sugar substitutes (though you could certainly make yours with raw honey if you prefer).

The last time I made this dish for a dinner party, I actually opted out of using the silicone molds and instead poured the entire mixture into a shallow, square glass baking dish and then placed it in the refrigerator for a couple of hours to set. Next, I cut it into squares while still in the dish, dumped the dish upside down so all the squares fell out, arranged the squares nicely on a serving platter, and then "dusted" them with a few generous spoonfuls of Primal Kitchen vanilla-coconut collagen fuel. The result was a gorgeous snow-kissed Turkish delight that my dinner guests "ooh-ed" and "ahh-ed" over, and that they couldn't seem to stop poking with a toothpick to grab yet another.

This recipe only takes about 15 to 20 minutes to whip up, with a brief chill afterward.

1. Mix the gelatin powder and ¼ cup cool water together in a small bowl and let the mixture sit for about 4 minutes so the gelatin can bloom.

2. Add the lemon juice, allulose, and (if desired) cinnamon to the thickened gelatin/water mixture.

3. Heat the apple cider vinegar and another ½ cup water in a small saucepan or pot over low heat until it is hot but not boiling.

4. Mix the apple cider vinegar and water with the gelatin mixture in the bowl and whisk or stir until the gelatin dissolves and all components are well mixed.

5. Pour it all into small silicone molds (or a baking dish; see description above) and refrigerate until set firmly, about 1 to 2 hours. If you're using a baking dish, cut the gummies into small squares, dust or sprinkle them with collagen powder, and serve with toothpicks.

*Yield:* 20 TO 24 GUMMIES

*Total Time:* 15 TO 20 MINUTES, PLUS 2 HOURS TO REFRIGERATE

## TOOLS AND MATERIALS

Small saucepan or pot

Small silicone molds (about the size of Reese's mini peanut butter cups is good) or square glass baking dish

## INGREDIENTS

3 tablespoon grass-fed gelatin powder

2 tablespoons lemon juice

2 to 3 tablespoons allulose

1 tablespoon Ceylon cinnamon (optional, for even more blood sugar control)

½ cup raw apple cider vinegar

2 tablespoons Primal Kitchen vanilla-coconut collagen fuel (optional)

**Note:** *I like the Great Lakes Wellness brand for a gelatin powder.*

# Chocolate Chai Gummies

Here's a fun edible twist on chai tea! The bonus: you will now know how to make your own homemade chai tea mix, which is great as a sipping beverage on a cold day, or served over ice with creamer and sweetener for a cool summer mocktail. Chai spices are incredibly high in antioxidants—anti-inflammatory and soreness-reducing compounds—and can help with blood sugar management, and you can easily take all the spices and spice ratios in the ingredients list below, add them to a large mason glass jar in whatever volume you'd like, and have them on hand for tea. I have to admit that the finished gummies themselves aren't half bad when paired with a bowl of coconut-vanilla ice cream too.

## INSTRUCTIONS FOR THE CHOCOLATE CHAI TEA MIX

1. Stir together all the powdered chai spice ingredients in a bowl.

## INSTRUCTIONS FOR THE GELATIN BITES

1. Pour the chocolate chai tea mix into the hot water in a small saucepan or pot on the stove and bring it to a boil. Lower the heat and allow the tea to simmer while you prepare the gelatin.

2. Add the gelatin to ¼ cup cool water in a separate bowl and allow it to dissolve completely, about 4 minutes.

3. Combine the spiced water with the gelatin/water mixture and whisk until mixed together.

4. Add the coconut milk and continue to stir.

5. Pour the mixture into small silicone molds and refrigerate until they set, about 35 to 40 minutes.

*Yield:* 20 TO 24 GUMMIES

*Total Time:* 15 TO 20 MINUTES, PLUS ABOUT 40 MINUTES TO REFRIGERATE

### TOOLS AND MATERIALS

Small saucepan or pot

Small silicone molds (about the size of Reese's mini peanut butter cups is good)

### INGREDIENTS FOR THE CHOCOLATE CHAI TEA MIX

2 teaspoons ground cardamom

2 teaspoons ground allspice

2 teaspoons ground nutmeg

4 teaspoons ground cinnamon

2 teaspoons ground cloves

4 teaspoons organic cacao powder

6 teaspoons ground ginger

### INGREDIENTS FOR THE GELATIN BITES

¾ cup hot water

3 tablespoons grass-fed gelatin

2 tablespoons full-fat coconut milk

**Note:** *Now that you know the basics, you can start off on your own culinary adventures with gelatin. The great thing about making gummies like this from gelatin is that you can modify them to suit your unique taste preferences, adding in any seasonings you prefer, such as turmeric, ginger, cinnamon, vanilla, or cacao!*

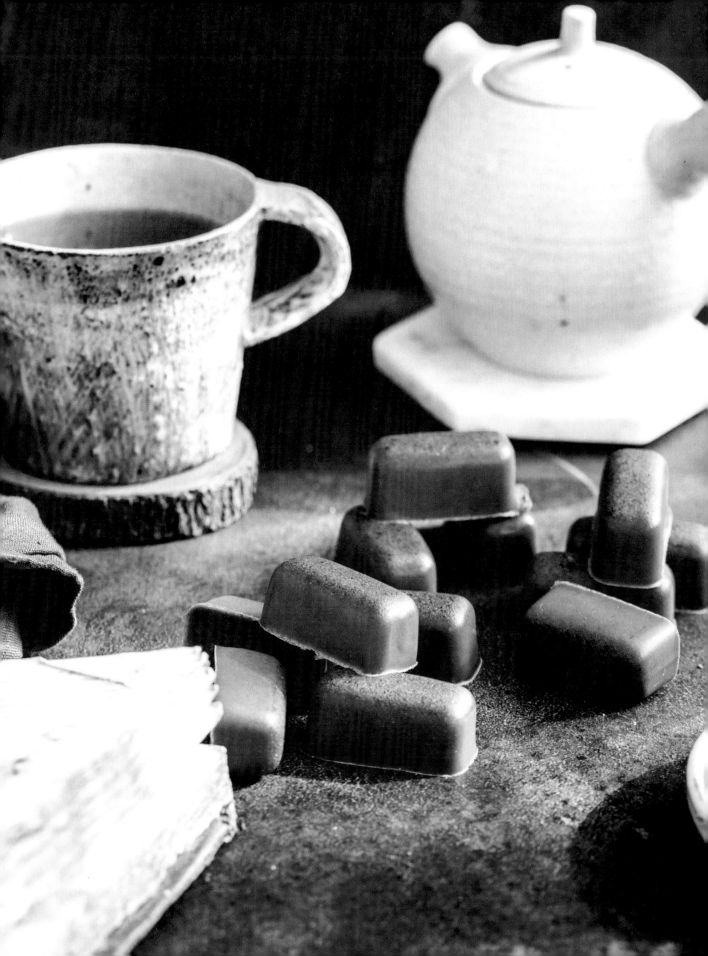

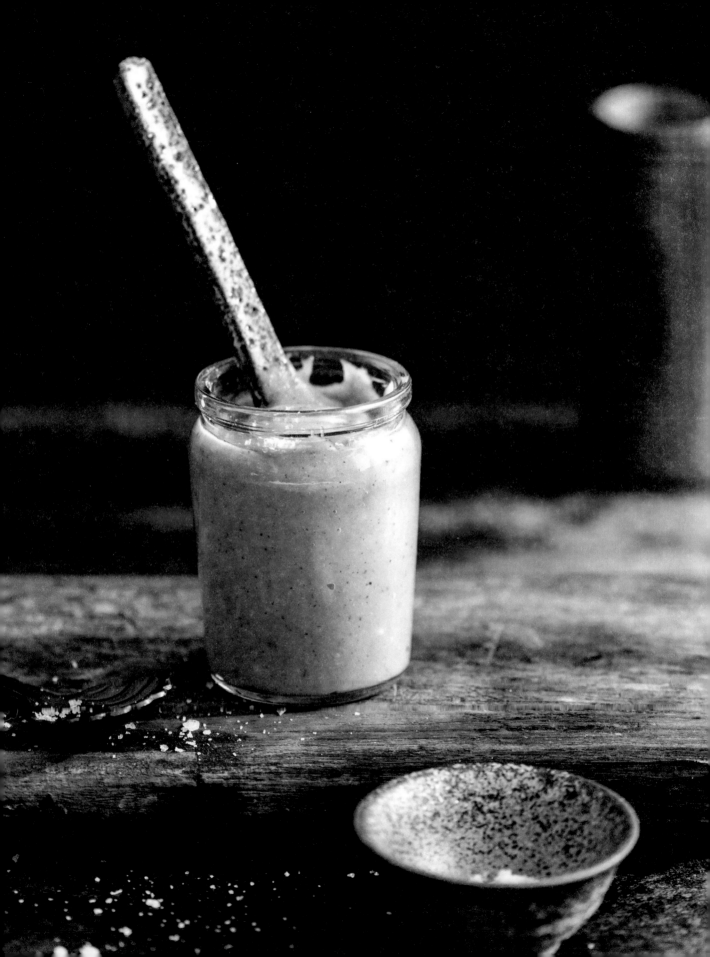

# Low-Carb Caramel Dipping Sauce

My sons originally prepared this healthy twist on caramel for their GoGreenfields podcast and YouTube cooking channel, and they love to occasionally make it now and serve it with any type of sliced fruit, particularly green apples, fresh peaches, or pears—though it's pretty good smeared on dark chocolate or dolloped atop ice cream too. In case you're watching your blood sugar levels, it has next to no net carbs per serving and is super easy to whip up quickly and serve as a simple dessert or appetizer.

1. Place the butter and allulose in a saucepan over medium-low heat. Heat the mixture until the butter melts and begins to bubble.

2. Lower the heat slightly and allow the mixture to simmer for 3 minutes while stirring occasionally.

3. Pour in the heavy cream and stir or whisk to mix. Then add the nut butter and salt and continue to stir or whisk to mix.

4. Reduce the heat to the lowest temperature and stir occasionally over next 8 to 12 minutes as mixture thickens. Pay attention to avoid any burning.

5. While the caramel is simmering, add ice cubes and water to a large mixing bowl to make an ice bath. Then, when the caramel has finished simmering, transfer the saucepan with the caramel in it to sit inside the large mixing bowl for 1 to 2 minutes. (If the caramel cools too much and splits, then simply transfer the pan back to the stovetop over low heat to warm it up again, stirring continuously. If you do this, you won't need to return the saucepan to the ice bath.)

6. Remove the saucepan from the ice bath and allow the sauce to set at room temperature to thicken, which takes 10 to 20 minutes.

7. When it's finished, it should be a thick and sticky caramel sauce that you can store in the refrigerator if you're not using it all at once (when you pull it from the fridge, you'll need to let it sit at room temperature for about 30 minutes to soften). Enjoy!

*Yield:* 6 TO 8 SERVINGS

*Total Time:* 30 TO 40 MINUTES

### TOOLS AND MATERIALS

A large mixing bowl with room to hold a saucepan

### INGREDIENTS

¼ cup butter

¼ cup allulose

½ cup heavy whipping cream or, if going dairy-free, coconut cream

1 teaspoon any nut butter of choice (almond or cashew butter works well)

1 teaspoon salt

Ice cubes and water (for ice bath)

# Buttered Maple Pecan Keto Brick Cheesecake Loaf

*Yield:* 8 TO 10 SERVINGS

*Total Time:* 60 MINUTES, PLUS OVERNIGHT REFRIGERATION

**TOOLS AND MATERIALS**

Cake mold, loaf pan, or baking pan

You've already learned about the amazing Keto Brick, which served as a tasty topping for the Keto-Vanilla-Blueberry Bowl (see page 110). But these things are versatile, good for more than just chopping and eating. You can actually melt down an entire Keto Brick to make some of the creamiest and most delicious cheesecake you'll ever have in your life. While I prefer the Buttered Maple Pecan flavor for this recipe, you may also want to experiment with Milk 'N Cookies, Peanut Butter, or Toasted Almond Coconut.

**INGREDIENTS FOR THE CRUST**

1 cup almond flour or coconut flour

½ Keto Brick, melted

½ teaspoon vanilla extract

2 tablespoons granulated sweetener

1 large egg

## INSTRUCTIONS FOR THE ALMOND FLOUR CRUST

1. Preheat the oven to 350°F.

2. Mix the almond flour with the melted half brick, vanilla, and sweetener. Add the egg and combine.

3. Spread this mixture onto a lightly greased cake mold, loaf pan, or baking pan, pressing it down with your fingers. Form a short lip around the pan. Bake the crust for 10 minutes.

4. Remove the crust from the oven and allow it to cool on the counter or in the fridge.

**INGREDIENTS FOR THE FILLING**

½ cup chopped pecans or walnuts

½ Keto Brick, melted

4 ounces cream cheese or coconut cream, room temperature

1 tablespoon sour cream, full-fat yogurt, or coconut yogurt

2 tablespoons monk fruit, allulose, or stevia

1 teaspoon maple or vanilla extract

1 large egg

Goji berries, blueberries, drizzled honey, low-sugar chocolate chips, or any other topping of your choice

## INSTRUCTIONS FOR THE FILLING

1. Preheat the oven to 350°F.

2. Sprinkle the pecans evenly over the cooled crust. Save a little extra for the topping if you want.

3. Mix the melted half brick, cream cheese, sour cream, monk fruit, maple extract, and egg (you can just mix this all up in the same pot you melted the brick in if you allow it to cool slightly so the egg doesn't cook).

4. Pour the filling over the crust and spread it evenly, ensuring that there are no exposed areas.

5. Bake for 20 to 25 minutes, or until the middle is set. Let the cheesecake loaf cool and then refrigerate, preferably overnight.

6. Sprinkle with toppings like the nuts reserved from step 2 or any of the toppings of your choice from the ingredients list. Cut the loaf into slices if you're using a loaf pan, or squares if you're using a brownie pan.

*Note:* *I melt the Keto Brick over low to medium heat in a pot on the stove top and stir frequently as it melts to keep it from burning, mostly because I'm too lazy to use a double boiler setup, which works even better.*

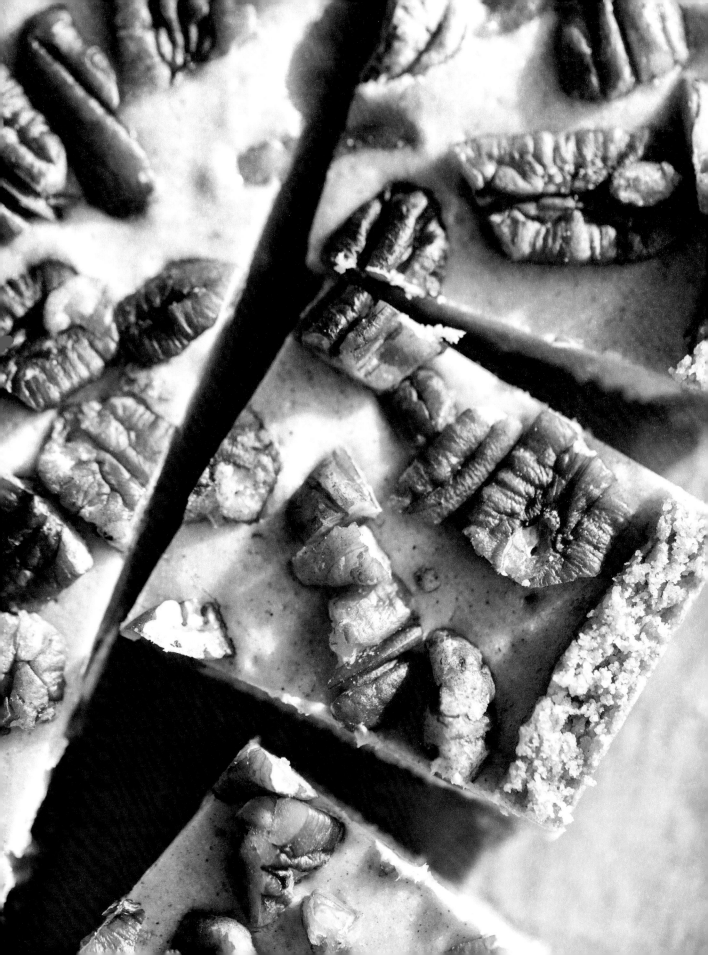

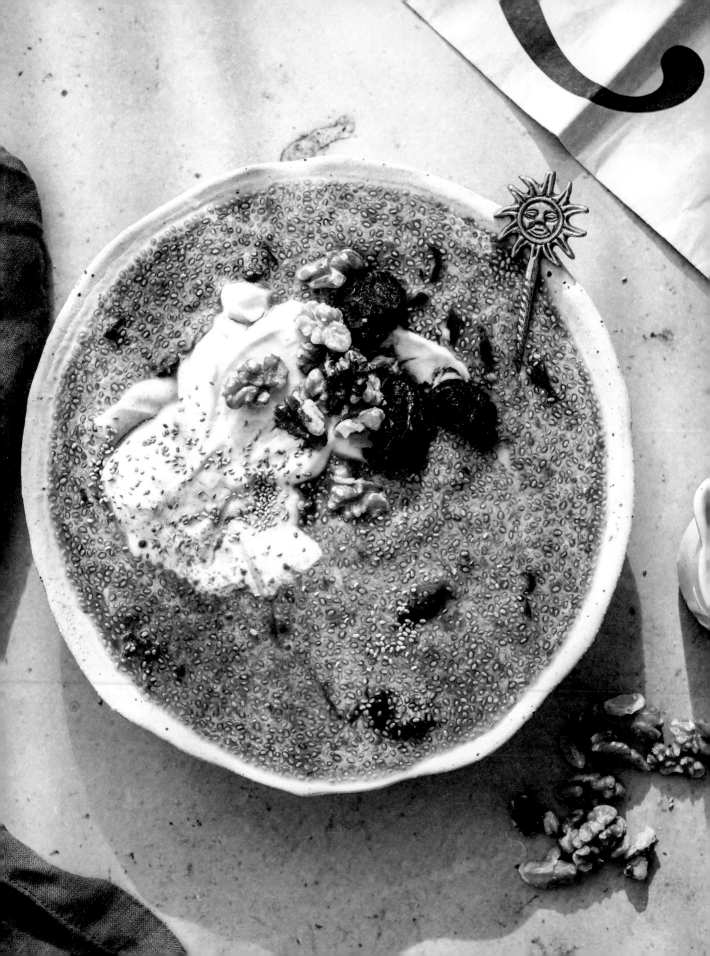

# Gut-Nourishing Chia Pudding

*Yield:* APPROXIMATELY 3 CUPS

*Total Time:* 10 TO 15 MINUTES TO PREPARE, 2 HOURS TO REFRIGERATE

## TOOLS AND MATERIALS

Large glass mason jar that holds at least 5 cups of liquid (needs to be about twice as many cups as the water you use because the pudding will expand)

## INGREDIENTS

½ cup chia seeds

2½ cups clean, pure filtered water

6 packets of Quinton Hypertonic

½ cup whole or chopped prunes

Honey, stevia, monk fruit, allulose, or any sweetener of your choice, to taste

*Note:* *Two to four heaping tablespoons of this before bed is quite satiating, but it's also wonderful to mix this blend with the Gut-Healing Super Yogurt for a tummy-friendly one-two combo.*

My friend and brilliant physician Dr. Matthew Cook—the "Dr. Strange" of medicine and a multi-time podcast guest of mine—turned me on to this simple variation of a chia pudding recipe that is incredibly nourishing to the gut, serves as a satiating, low-calorie, low-carbohydrate nighttime snack, and—brace yourself—when taken as a nighttime snack, alleviates morning constipation. The secret sauce in this recipe is the addition of Quinton minerals, one of the most complete electrolyte sources on the planet, and bowel-moving prunes, which also happen to be an excellent source of vitamins, minerals, fiber, and antioxidants.

Most recipes call for a 1:10 ratio of chia seeds to water for a chia seed pudding, but I like my pudding nice and thick, so I actually use a 1:5 ratio and simply stir a bit longer and more completely to ensure all the chia seeds are soaked. You can always use less chia seed if you want your pudding less thick.

1. Add the chia seeds, water, and Quinton to a large mason jar and stir, mix, and/or shake to ensure that all the chia seeds are completely covered in water. There shouldn't be any clumps left.

2. Add the prunes and stir them in completely.

3. Drizzle in the honey to taste and stir completely again.

4. Cover and refrigerate the pudding for at least 2 hours or overnight.

# Sweet Chicken Pudding

*Yield:* 8 TO 10 SERVINGS

*Total Time:* 65 MINUTES PLUS
6 HOURS TO REFRIGERATE

**TOOLS AND MATERIALS**

Fine mesh strainer

Hand blender

**INGREDIENTS**

2 medium-to-large chicken breasts

4 cups coconut milk, almond milk, or oat milk

⅓ cup non-GMO cornstarch

⅓ cup white rice flour or any other gluten-free flour

½ cup honey, plus more for drizzling

1 teaspoon vanilla extract

1 teaspoon cinnamon

1 teaspoon ground nutmeg

Raisins (optional, for topping)

**Note:** *Coconut milk is best for this recipe, as it's the most fatty and creamy, but if you aren't avoiding dairy, you can use whole milk or even heavy cream.*

During one of our Greenfield family Iron Chef competitions (see page 53), the mystery ingredient was chicken. The rules required me to make a unique chicken entrée and appetizer. I also had to come up with some kind of a chicken-based dessert. So I modified a traditional Turkish dessert with a few of my own twists and came up with sweet chicken pudding that was surprisingly delightful, didn't taste anything like chicken breast, and served as a high-protein snack I kept in the fridge and dove into for several days after the competition. It's great served on its own drizzled with honey and sprinkled with raisins or dried berries and also quite good served with crunchy rice crackers for dipping.

1. Place the chicken in a saucepan with enough water to cover it. Bring the water to a boil and cook the chicken well. Thin breasts will cook in about 8 minutes; large chicken breasts will need up to 15 minutes. The chicken is done when it registers 165°F in the thickest part of the meat with an instant-read thermometer. You can also cut into the chicken to see if it's cooked through.

2. Transfer the cooked chicken from the saucepan to a bowl. Pull the meat apart with your fingers or use a fork to separate it into fine strips. Continue to shred the chicken as finely as you can.

3. Cool the chicken by putting all the chicken shreds into a bowl of ice water for about 20 minutes. Then strain out the water using a fine mesh strainer.

4. Put the coconut milk in a large saucepan and boil it for 5 minutes. Add the cold shredded chicken to the milk and blend the milk and chicken with a hand blender until very smooth. Return the pan to the heat and continue to cook for about 20 minutes more, stirring occasionally.

5. In a separate bowl, whisk together the cornstarch, rice flour, and about 2 cups of water until smooth. Remove the milk from the heat. Using your whisk, drizzle the starch in a very fine stream into the milk as you whisk it.

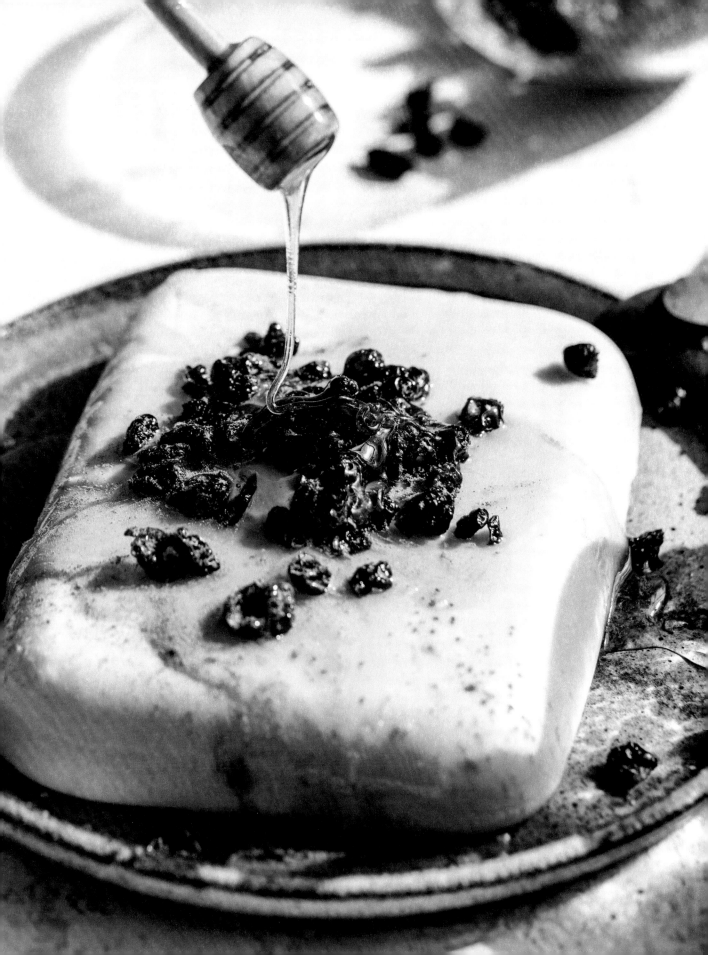

**6.** Once all the starch is whisked in, return the pan to the heat and bring it to just below boiling temperature while stirring constantly. Cook for about 5 minutes until it begins to thicken.

**7.** Stir in the honey and vanilla extract and cook for another 15 minutes, continuing to stir occasionally (I like a thick wooden spoon for this because it's going to get pretty hard to stir). The pudding should become so thick that you can no longer easily stir it.

**8.** Wet the bottom and sides of a shallow glass tray or casserole dish. Spoon the pudding into the wet tray and let it cool down to room temperature. Then cover and refrigerate it for about 6 hours.

**9.** To serve, you can cut your pudding with a knife or pie server, or scoop it out with a large spoon. Sprinkle some cinnamon and raisins, if using, and then drizzle more honey on each portion prior to serving.

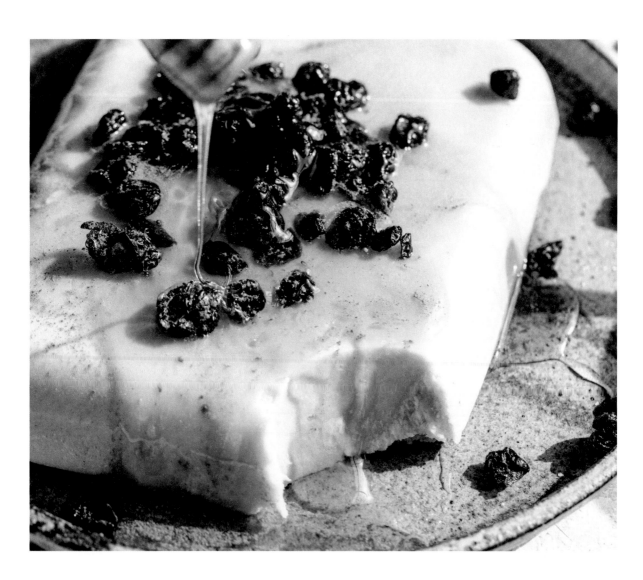

# Resources

Visit BoundlessKitchen.com/resources for even more information on the resources listed here and throughout the book.

## Books

*The 4-Hour Chef* by Timothy Ferriss

*Anti-Factory Farm Shopping Guide* by Evgeny Trufkin

*Boundless: Upgrade Your Brain, Optimize Your Body & Defy Aging* by Ben Greenfield

*Boundless Cookbook* by Ben Greenfield

*The Complete Guide to Hunting, Butchering, and Cooking Wild Game* by Steven Rinella

*The Good Life: Lessons from the World's Longest Scientific Study of Happiness* by Robert Waldinger, M.D., and Marc Schulz, Ph.D.

*The Longevity Solution* by Dr. James DiNicolantonio

*The Obesity Fix* by Dr. James DiNicolantonio

*Super Gut* by William Davis, M.D.

*The Wildatarian Diet* by Teri Cochrane

## Podcasts

"Why You Shouldn't Let Modern Baby Food Anywhere Near Your Baby (& What to Use Instead to Make Your Baby Stronger & Smarter)," *BenGreenfieldLife*, August 31, 2019

"The Ultimate Vinegar Extravaganza," *BenGreenfieldLife*, February 18, 2023

Why Wild-Caught Fish Isn't Necessarily Better," *BenGreenfieldLife*, October 9, 2021

## Websites

Captain's Fine Foods, captainsfinefoods.com

Cultures for Health, culturesforhealth.com

Cutting Edge Cultures, cuttingedgecultures.com

Dry Farm Wines, dryfarmwines.com

Eatwild, eatwild.com

Fossil Farms, fossilfarms.com

Fresh-Pressed Olive Oil Club, freshpressedoliveoil.com

Greene Prairie Shrimp, greeneprairieaquafarm.com

Henry & Lisa's Natural Seafood, ecofish.com

Kettle & Fire, kettleandfire.com

MrBreakfast.com

Organifi Red Juice, organifishop.com

Schiff, schiffvitamins.com

SeafoodWatch.org

Seatopia, seatopia.fish

Selva Shrimp, selvashrimp.com

*Sous Vide Everything*, youtube.com/@SousVideEverything

The Spruce Eats, thespruceeats.com

Thrive Market, thrivemarket.com

US Wellness Meats, grasslandbeef.com

White Oak Pastures, whiteoakpastures.com

Whole Foods, wholefoodsmarket.com

Wild Idea Buffalo Company, wildideabuffalo.com

## Kitchen Tools, Materials, and Equipment

Air fryer (Cuisinart or Breville)

Amber glass bottle

Baking sheet

Blender

Blowtorch

Bowl

Box-style cheese grater

Cast-iron skillet

Cheesecloth

Circular springform pan

Cocktail shaker

Coffee filter

Colander or mesh strainer

Dutch oven

Food dehydrator

Food processor

FoodSaver bags

Frothing wand

Glass mason jars

Grill (Traeger)

Jars

Kore

Mandoline

Meat thermometer

Multi-cooker (Breville)

Oil thermometer

Oven

Parchment paper

Popsicle molds

Pressure cooker (Breville, Ninja, or Instant Pot)

Pyrex glass container

Roasting pan or broiling pan

Rubber bands

Silicone donut molds

Silicone freezer molds

Slow cooker

Sous vide bag

Sous vide cooker (Anova)

Sous vide joule

Springform cake pan

Square baking dish

Stasher bag

Stasher bag (large)

Thermometer

Toothpicks

Waffle iron

Whisk

Yogurt maker

## Pantry items

100-proof vodka

Allspice

Allulose

Almond flour

Almond milk (unsweetened)

Angelica Mill Himalayan Tartary Buckwheat Flour

Apple cider vinegar

Arrowroot powder

Ashwagandha (powdered or liquid)

Avocado oil

Avocado oil spray

Baking soda

Balsamic vinegar

Barùka Butter

Barùkas Trail Mix

Bee pollen

Big Bold Health Himalayan Tartary Buckwheat Flour

Biodynamic wine (Dry Farm Wines)

Black pepper

Bob's Red Mill Coconut Flour

Bob's Red Mill Gluten-Free Flour

Bob's Red Mill Tapioca Starch

Bone broth

Butter (grass-fed, grass-finished, such as Kerrygold)

Buttermilk (organic)

Cacao powder (organic)

Calamansi gourmet vinegar

Cardamom

Ceylon cinnamon

Chia seeds

Chili powder

Cinnamon stick

Coconut cream

Coconut flakes

Coconut flour (Bob's Red Mill)

Coconut milk

Coconut sugar

Coconut water

Cornstarch

Dr. Thomas Cowan's vegetable powders

Dried elderberries

Dried elderflowers

Duck fat

Extra-virgin olive oil

Garlic powder

Ghee

Gluten-free flour (Bob's Red Mill)

Goat's milk

Grass-fed gelatin powder

Guar gum

Herbes de Provence seasoning (organic)

Himalayan Tartary Buckwheat Flour (Angelica Mill or Big Bold Health)

Honey

Inulin powder

Joey's Hot Sauce

Kerrygold butter

Ketchup

Kion Clean Energy Bar

Kion Clean Protein

Lard

Macadamia nut oil

Medjool dates

Monk fruit

Nutmeg powder

Omica Organics Stevia (plain or butterscotch)

Onion powder

Paprika

Parmigiano-Reggiano cheese

Peanut oil

Pear balsamic vinegar

Powdered mushrooms (Four Sigmatic Mushrooms, particularly Cordyceps, Chaga, Lion's Mane, and 10-Mushroom Blend)

Powdered sugar (organic)

Powdered vanilla-flavored ketones (Perfect Keto Vanilla Flavor)

Primal Kitchen Buffalo Sauce

Primal Kitchen Golden BBQ Sauce

Primal Kitchen Mustard

Primal Kitchen Vanilla Coconut Collagen Fuel

Probiotic powder/yogurt starter

Raw honey

Red pepper

Red wine

Reishi extract

Rice bran oil

Roasted almonds

Salt (table, Himalayan, sea salt, kona)

Sea vegetable powder

Sesame oil

Shiso leaves

Spirulina powder

Stevia (Omica Organics plain or butterscotch)

Sugar

Sweetener (monk fruit sweetener or agave syrup)

Tallow

T. J. Robinson's artisan vinegars

Tapioca powder

Tapioca starch (Bob's Red Mill)

Tortillas

Vanilla extract

Vegetable powders (Dr. Thomas Cowan's)

Vinegar (T. J. Robinson's artisan vinegars)

Walnut oil

Walnuts

Water kefir grains

Worcestershire sauce

## Supplements

*Bacillus coagulans* GBI-30,6086 (Thorne)

Charcoal pills/powder

Chocolate whey protein (Kion Clean Protein)

CoenzymeQ10 (CoQ10)

Colostrum (Kion)

Element Health Maximum Strength CBD

Flavored electrolytes (Protekt watermelon or LMNT citrus salt flavors)

Folate

Glycine

Hydrogen tablets

Jigsaw Adrenal Health Cocktail

Keto Brick

KetoneIQ or KetoneAid Ke4

Kion Aminos

Kion Colostrum

Kion Creatine (or Thorne)

Kion Vanilla Whey Protein

*Lactobacillus gasseri* BNR17

*Lactobacillus reuteri*

Lecithin

LMNT (electrolyte powder)

Manna

Protekt

Quicksilver Scientific Liposomal GABA with L-Theanine

Quinton Isotonic

Quinton Hypertonic

Serenity Kids Berry Butternut Dairy-Free Smoothie + Protein

Schiff Digestive Advantage

Thorne Bacillus Coagulans

## Meat, Fish, and Chicken

Beef tongue

Braunschweiger

Canned Oregon pink shrimp

Fish collar

Liverwurst

Organ meat

Pasture-raised pork

Wild game roast (venison, mutton, elk, bison, moose)

## A NOTE ON PROTEIN SOURCES

I've only scratched the surface of the importance of choosing high-quality and well-balanced protein sources in this book. I get into plenty more detail in my book *Boundless: Upgrade Your Brain, Optimize Your Body & Defy Aging.*

But let's say you're at least convinced by now that you don't need to eat just lettuce and carrots for the rest of your life. Where can you get high-quality meat these days that satisfies the criteria of grass-fed, grass-finished animals grown in a regenerative, sustainable, ethical manner?

A few of my favorite sources include:

• **Thrive Market:** 100 percent grass-fed, pasture-raised beef shipped right to your door. All of their beef comes from Osorno, Chile, where grass is abundant and the climate is ideal for letting cows graze outdoors year-round. No chemicals, artificial fertilizers, or antibiotics are used. Low-density grazing methods are used to maintain the integrity of the precious land and soil. thrivemarket.com

• **US Wellness Meats** (use code GREENFIELD for a 15 percent store-wide discount): Tender and tasty, without all the excess fat of animals fed with grain in confinement. Full of nutrients that can only come from a fully grass-fed diet—omega-3 fatty acids, vitamin A, vitamin E, and CLA (conjugated linoleic acids)—and free of all the pesticides, hormones, and antibiotics that are found in grain-fed beef. grasslandbeef.com

• **White Oak Pastures:** Grass-fed beef, goat, and lamb and pastured chicken, duck, goose, and more. Animals are raised in a regenerative manner using humane animal management practices. whiteoakpastures.com

• **Eatwild:** The number one clearinghouse for information about pasture-based farming and features a state-by-state plus Canada directory of local farmers who sell their pastured farm and ranch products directly to consumers. eatwild.com

• **Seatopia:** In my podcast "Why Wild-Caught Fish Isn't Necessarily Better, the Truth About Farmed Fish, How to Get Guilt-Free, Gourmet Seafood, Delicious DIY Sushi & Sashimi Recipes & Much More!," I teach you about Seatopia, which makes eating and exploring truly sustainable gourmet seafood easier and more fun by delivering award-winning seafood direct from artisan regenerative farms right to your doorstep, all in 100 percent plastic-free and Styrofoam-free packaging—100 percent transparency, 100 percent sushi-grade, 100 percent antibiotic-free, certified sustainable, and mercury-free. Plus each shipment includes QR code–scannable recipes from celebrity and Michelin-starred chefs. seatopia.fish

## A SPECIAL NOTE ON SHRIMP

In addition to seafood suppliers such as Seatopia, many grocery stores sell wild or local shrimp from clean waters, which is important because *Consumer Reports* has reported that farm-raised or foreign shrimp is more likely to have antibiotics that you shouldn't eat. You can ask your fishmonger or butcher at the grocery store whether the shrimp has indeed been treated with the preservatives mentioned on page 67.

There are actually over 3,000 species of shrimp, but only four shrimp options are currently considered sustainable—meaning they are caught or farmed with minimal environmental impact: pink shrimp from Oregon (best choice on the fantastic Seafood Watch list); spot prawns from the Pacific Northwest; brown, white, and pink shrimp from the Gulf of Mexico (except Louisiana); and shrimp from U.S. and Canadian waters in the northern Atlantic. You can also look for two logos that certify shrimp were farmed sustainably: the Global Aquaculture Alliance's blue fish logo or the Aquaculture Stewardship Council's logo.

Wild Planet also has a fresh-flavored, clean, and sustainable canned Oregon pink shrimp. Other brands vetted by retailers such as Whole Foods or a third party like Seafood Watch, both of which enforce rigorous standards on suppliers, include Selva Shrimp, Henry & Lisa's Natural Seafood, Captain's Fine Foods, and Greene Prairie Shrimp Farm.

## FATS AND OILS

Choosing the right fat for cooking is important for both good health and good flavor. Once a fat is heated past its "smoke point," it starts to break down, releasing free radicals and other harmful compounds and making your food taste burned and bitter. Use the table below to find the ideal fat for whatever delicious dish you're whipping up.

| FAT / OIL | SMOKE POINT (UNREFINED/REFINED) | BEST USES |
|---|---|---|
| Avocado oil | 520°F | • high-heat cooking<br>• low-heat cooking<br>• dressing<br>• finishing |
| Butter, ghee | 300/480°F | • high-heat cooking<br>• baking |
| Coconut oil | 350/450°F | • high-heat cooking<br>• sautéing<br>• baking |
| Duck fat | 375°F | • high-heat cooking |
| Lard (pork, bacon fat) | 375°F | • high-heat cooking |
| Macadamia nut oil | 410°F | • low-heat cooking<br>• dressing<br>• finishing |
| Olive oil | 320/465°F | • high-heat cooking<br>• low-heat cooking<br>• dressing<br>• finishing |
| Peanut oil | 230/450°F | • high-heat cooking |
| Rice bran oil | 415°F | • low-heat cooking |
| Sesame oil | 450°F | • dressing<br>• finishing |
| Tallow (beef fat) | 400°F | • high-heat cooking |
| Walnut oil | 400°F | • dressing<br>• finishing |

# References

Bickford, Paula C., Jun Tan, R. Douglas Shytle, Cyndy D. Sanberg, Nagwa El-Badri, and Paul R. Sanberg. "Nutraceuticals Synergistically Promote Proliferation of Human Stem Cells." *Stem Cells and Development* 15, no. 1 (February 2006): 118–23. https://doi.org/10.1089/scd.2006.15.118.

Carlsen, Monica H., Bente L. Halvorsen, Kari Holte, Siv K Bøhn, Steinar Dragland, Laura Sampson, Carol Willey, et al. "The Total Antioxidant Content of More Than 3100 Foods, Beverages, Spices, Herbs and Supplements Used Worldwide." *Nutrition Journal* 9, no. 1 (January 22, 2010). https://doi.org/10.1186/1475-2891-9-3.

Crabtree, Christopher D., Thanh Blade, Parker N. Hyde, Alex Buga, Madison L. Kackley, Teryn N. Sapper, Oishika Panda, et al. "Bis Hexanoyl (R)-1,3-Butanediol, a Novel Ketogenic Ester, Acutely Increases Circulating r- and s-ß-Hydroxybutyrate Concentrations in Healthy Adults." *Journal of the American Nutrition Association* 42, no. 2 (February 2023): 169–77. https://doi.org/10.1080/07315724.2021.2015476.

Dafni, Amots, Saleh Aqil Khatib, and Guillermo Benítez. "The Doctrine of Signatures in Israel—Revision and Spatiotemporal Patterns." *Plants* 10, no. 7 (July 1, 2021): 1346. https://doi.org/10.3390/plants10071346.

"The Earliest Alcoholic Beverage in the World." Research, Penn Museum. https://www.penn.museum/research/project.php?pid=12#:~:text=Chemical%20analyses%20recently%20confirmed%20that,in%20the%20Yellow%20River%20Valley.

Ershoff, B. H. "Beneficial Effect of Liver Feeding on Swimming Capacity of Rats in Cold Water." *Experimental Biology and Medicine* 77, no. 3 (July 1951): 488–91. https://doi.org/10.3181/00379727-77-18824.

"How Safe Is Your Shrimp?" *Consumer Reports*, April 24, 2015. https://www.consumerreports.org/cro/magazine/2015/06/shrimp-safety/index.htm.

Kitada, Munehiro, Yoshio Ogura, Itaru Monno, Jing Xu, and Daisuke Koya. "Effect of Methionine Restriction on Aging: Its Relationship to Oxidative Stress." *Biomedicines* 9, no. 2 (January 29, 2021): 130. https://doi.org/10.3390/biomedicines9020130.

Spreadbury, Ian. "Comparison with Ancestral Diets Suggests Dense Acellular Carbohydrates Promote an Inflammatory Microbiota, and May Be the Primary Dietary Cause of Leptin Resistance and Obesity." *Diabetes, Metabolic Syndrome and Obesity: Targets and Therapy* 5 (July 6, 2012): 175–89. https://doi.org/10.2147/dmso.s33473.

# Conversion Chart

| Standard Cup | Fine Powder (e.g., flour) | Grain (e.g., rice) | Granular (e.g., sugar) | Liquid Solids (e.g., butter) | Liquid (e.g., milk) |
|---|---|---|---|---|---|
| 1 | 140 g | 150 g | 190 g | 200 g | 240 ml |
| ¾ | 105 g | 113 g | 143 g | 150 g | 180 ml |
| ⅔ | 93 g | 100 g | 125 g | 133 g | 160 ml |
| ½ | 70 g | 75 g | 95 g | 100 g | 120 ml |
| ⅓ | 47 g | 50 g | 63 g | 67 g | 80 ml |
| ¼ | 35 g | 38 g | 48 g | 50 g | 60 ml |
| ⅛ | 18 g | 19 g | 24 g | 25 g | 30 ml |

| Useful Equivalents for Cooking/Oven Temperatures | | | |
|---|---|---|---|
| Process | Fahrenheit | Celsius | Gas Mark |
| Freeze Water | 32° F | 0° C | |
| Room Temperature | 68° F | 20° C | |
| Boil Water | 212° F | 100° C | |
| Bake | 325° F | 160° C | 3 |
| | 350° F | 180° C | 4 |
| | 375° F | 190° C | 5 |
| | 400° F | 200° C | 6 |
| | 425° F | 220° C | 7 |
| | 450° F | 230° C | 8 |
| Broil | | | Grill |

| Useful Equivalents for Liquid Ingredients by Volume | | | | |
|---|---|---|---|---|
| ¼ tsp | | | | 1 ml |
| ½ tsp | | | | 2 ml |
| 1 tsp | | | | 5 ml |
| 3 tsp | 1 tbsp | | ½ fl oz | 15 ml |
| | 2 tbsp | ⅛ cup | 1 fl oz | 30 ml |
| | 4 tbsp | ¼ cup | 2 fl oz | 60 ml |
| | 5⅓ tbsp | ⅓ cup | 3 fl oz | 80 ml |
| | 8 tbsp | ½ cup | 4 fl oz | 120 ml |
| | 10⅔ tbsp | ⅔ cup | 5 fl oz | 160 ml |
| | 12 tbsp | ¾ cup | 6 fl oz | 180 ml |
| | 16 tbsp | 1 cup | 8 fl oz | 240 ml |
| | 1 pt | 2 cups | 16 fl oz | 480 ml |
| | 1 qt | 4 cups | 32 fl oz | 960 ml |

| Useful Equivalents for Dry Ingredients by Weight | | |
|---|---|---|
| (To convert ounces to grams, multiply the number of ounces by 30.) | | |
| 1 oz | 1/16 lb | 30 g |
| 4 oz | ¼ lb | 120 g |
| 8 oz | ½ lb | 240 g |
| 12 oz | ¾ lb | 360 g |
| 16 oz | 1 lb | 480 g |

| Useful Equivalents for Length | | | | |
|---|---|---|---|---|
| (To convert inches to centimeters, multiply the number of inches by 2.5.) | | | | |
| 1 in | | | 2.5 cm | |
| 6 in | ½ ft | | 15 cm | |
| 12 in | 1 ft | | 30 cm | |
| 36 in | 3 ft | 1 yd | 90 cm | |
| 40 in | | | 100 cm | 1 m |

# INDEX

## Also by Ben Greenfield

*Beyond Training*
*Boundless*
*Boundless Cookbook*
*Boundless Parenting*
*Endure*
*Fit Soul*

**Ben Greenfield** is a health consultant, speaker, and *New York Times* best-selling author of a wide variety of books, including *Beyond Training, Boundless, Fit Soul, Boundless Cookbook, Endure*, and *Boundless Parenting Book*. Ben is a frequent contributor to health and wellness publications and websites and a highly sought-after speaker, and his understanding of functional exercise, nutrition, and the delicate balance between performance and health has helped thousands of people around the world achieve their goals and improve their quality of life.

Ben is an advisor, investor, and board member of multiple corporations in the health and fitness industry and is also the co-founder of KION, a nutritional supplements company that combines time-honored superfoods with modern science to allow human beings to achieve peak performance, defy aging, and live an adventurous, fulfilling, joyful, and limitless life. Via online, phone, e-mail, and in-person consulting,

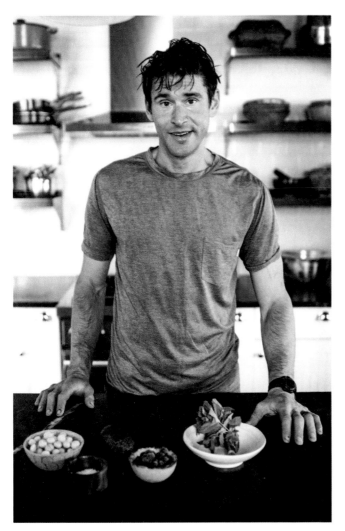

Ben coaches and trains individuals all over the world for health, longevity, and performance. He also works with corporations and teams for body and brain performance enhancement, specializing in productivity, faith, family, fat loss, digestion, brain, sleep, hormone, anti-aging, parenting, relationships, mental performance, and overall wellness for achieving an optimized life. As a public speaker on longevity, anti-aging, biohacking, fitness, nutrition, cognition, positive psychology, motivation, and spirituality, Ben has hosted several top-ranked fitness and health podcasts, including most notably the *Ben Greenfield Life* show.

Ben's mission is to serve those who, like himself, desire to live life to the fullest, experience deep meaning, purpose, happiness, fulfillment, and connection, explore and enjoy every nook and cranny of God's great creation, and discover how to achieve full optimization of mind, body, and spirit with boundless energy. Ben lives in the Inland Northwest with his wife, Jessa, and their twin sons, River and Terran, where he exercises, enjoys fiction, guitar, ukulele, spearfishing, bowhunting, pickleball, plant foraging, cooking, and savoring all of God's creation.

@bengreenfieldfitness on IG

https://www.facebook.com/BGFitness

We hope you enjoyed this Hay House book. If you'd like to receive our online catalog featuring additional information on Hay House books and products, or if you'd like to find out more about the Hay Foundation, please contact:

Hay House, Inc., P.O. Box 5100, Carlsbad, CA 92018-5100
(760) 431-7695 or (800) 654-5126
(760) 431-6948 (fax) or (800) 650-5115 (fax)
www.hayhouse.com® • www.hayfoundation.org

———

*Published in Australia by:* Hay House Australia Pty. Ltd.,
18/36 Ralph St., Alexandria NSW 2015
*Phone:* 612-9669-4299 • *Fax:* 612-9669-4144
www.hayhouse.com.au

*Published in the United Kingdom by:* Hay House UK, Ltd.,
The Sixth Floor, Watson House, 54 Baker Street, London W1U 7BU
*Phone:* +44 (0)20 3927 7290 • *Fax:* +44 (0)20 3927 7291
www.hayhouse.co.uk

*Published in India by:* Hay House Publishers India,
Muskaan Complex, Plot No. 3, B-2, Vasant Kunj, New Delhi 110 070
*Phone:* 91-11-4176-1620 • *Fax:* 91-11-4176-1630
www.hayhouse.co.in

———

## Access New Knowledge.
## Anytime. Anywhere.

Learn and evolve at your own pace
with the world's leading experts.

www.hayhouseU.com

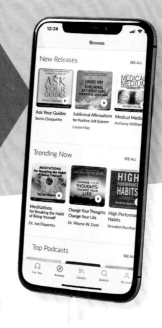
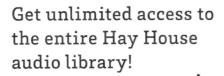

# Hay House Podcasts
## Bring Fresh, Free Inspiration Each Week!

Hay House proudly offers a selection of life-changing audio content via our most popular podcasts!

### Hay House Meditations Podcast

Features your favorite Hay House authors guiding you through meditations designed to help you relax and rejuvenate. Take their words into your soul and cruise through the week!

### Dr. Wayne W. Dyer Podcast

Discover the timeless wisdom of Dr. Wayne W. Dyer, world-renowned spiritual teacher and affectionately known as "the father of motivation." Each week brings some of the best selections from the 10-year span of Dr. Dyer's talk show on Hay House Radio.

### Hay House Podcast

Enjoy a selection of insightful and inspiring lectures from Hay House Live events, listen to some of the best moments from previous Hay House Radio episodes, and tune in for exclusive interviews and behind-the-scenes audio segments featuring leading experts in the fields of alternative health, self-development, intuitive medicine, success, and more! Get motivated to live your best life possible by subscribing to the free Hay House Podcast.

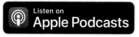

*Find Hay House podcasts on iTunes, or visit www.HayHouse.com/podcasts for more info.*

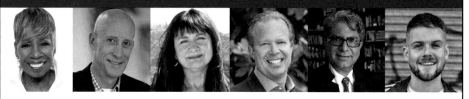